Dry All Night

Also by Alison Mack

TOILET LEARNING: The Picture Book Technique for Children and Parents

Dry All Night

The Picture Book Technique
That Stops Bedwetting

by

ALISON MACK

Pictures by Miriam Tobias

Foreword by David Wilensky, M.D.
Fellow of the American Academy of Pediatrics

LITTLE, BROWN AND COMPANY
BOSTON   TORONTO   LONDON

FIRST EDITION

Library of Congress Cataloging-in-Publication Data

Mack, Alison.
    Dry all night / Alison Mack.
        p.   cm.
    Summary: A step-by-step program for curing bedwetting, with separate sections for parent and child.
    ISBN 0-316-54226-1
    [1. Bedwetting.]   I. Title.
    RJ476.E6M33   1989
    618.92′849 — dc19   88-32524
                                      CIP
                                      AC

10 9 8 7 6 5 4 3 2 1

RRD OH

Published simultaneously in Canada
by Little, Brown & Company (Canada) Limited
PRINTED IN THE UNITED STATES OF AMERICA

This book is dedicated to
my mother
and
my father

Contents

Foreword

ENURESIS, or bedwetting, is one of the most common and troublesome conditions found in school-age children. A substantial proportion of them may suffer from occasional or frequent wetting at night. This problem can have significant psychological fallout: loss of self-esteem, heightened tension between parents and children, experiential constrictions (e.g., embarrassment at sleeping at a friend's house or going camping), and peer rejection are common sequelae.

The possible reasons for bedwetting are numerous, and consultation with one's family physician or pediatrician is in order before starting on any treatment program. In the vast majority of cases, however, no medical problem will be present.

This book, by the author of the classic *Toilet Learning: The Picture Book Technique for Children and Parents,* offers a promising solution for these many children. The beauty of its approach is, firstly, in the fulfillment of the medical dictum *primum non nocere* — "in the first place, do no harm!" It involves no side effects, such as are associated with drug therapy for enuresis. It requires no special equipment or complicated demands on other family members.

Secondly, success will be the result of the child's own efforts. The result will be a sense of mastery that will correct for the decline in self-esteem so often found in the enuretic child. The appealing format of *Dry All Night* provides an elegant, yet simple, step-by-step program that can be easily implemented, eliminating the negative familial interaction so commonly found in cases of enuresis, and creating a new positive union between parent and child.

David Wilensky, M.D.
Fellow of the American Academy of Pediatrics

Acknowledgments

CREATING THIS BOOK was especially rewarding to me because it was a family project. My son Max conceptualized key illustrations and was master of the photocopying machine as, during the development process, successive versions metamorphosed. My daughter Rose helped me hone the text of Part 2 for ease of comprehension, and made the Dry All Night scoreboard that appears there. My son Sam stood v-e-r-y still while being sketched as the model for Christopher. My daughter Goldie cooperated by having just enough accidents to enable me to evaluate materials for keeping bedding dry. My husband processed my words with the help of an elf from Orem, Utah, named WordPerfect. My father was his usual resourceful self in obtaining the unobtainable, yesterday. And my father-in-law's tireless efforts in supplying me with research materials included the not-easy task of persuading the manager of the local school bus company that his motive in photographing one of their vehicles from every possible angle was entirely benign.

My thanks to Miriam Tobias, to whom I hope this book will be a source of enduring satisfaction.

The conversations I had with Professor Marco Caine, M.D., F.R.C.S., Head, Department of Urology, Hadassah University Medical Center; Mordecai Halperin, M.D., of Shaarei Tzedek Medical Center; and Paul R. Silverstein, M.D., F.A.C.S., of the Berkshire Urological Office, regarding the urodynamics of enuresis, were illuminating. One of the most gratifying moments during the course of my research was when I described the Dry All Night method to Professor Caine, and he responded, "Ah — so the book is the therapist!"

I thank Joel D. Curran, M.D., F.A.A.P., for discussing his approach to enuresis with me. I valued the reservations expressed to me by Lazar Fruchter, M.D., F.A.A.P., A.B.A.I., regarding an etiological role for food sensitivities in enuresis. William Josephs, Ph.D., a psychologist of remarkable insight, gave me the benefit of his expertise in the clinical use of guided imagery. And I am indebted to Eli E. Lasch, M.D., M.P.H., for having taught me that every disorder of the body is a lesson.

Special thanks are due to Rivka Rakov. With her accurate eye, her direct tongue, her love of children's books, and her love of children, she contributed inestimably to this book.

Mickie Klugman played a vital role in the development of Part 2 and drew and lettered the Dry All Night scoreboard that appears in Part 1. Judith Abinun was generous in permitting me to use the equipment of her graphic art studio. Galit Stein and Ariel Ullmann of Mamsheet Camel Farm were warm hosts. Keiko and Shigeo Yamada double-checked my Japanese.

Dr. and Mrs. Martin Dann shared their experiences with me. Charles S. Kazan, in ably assisting with library research, saw chains where another might have perceived only links. R. Matis Weinberg, teacher, and father of nine, gave wise counsel.

Dr. Roger Broughton, of the University of Ottawa School of Medicine Division of Neurology; Dr. Edmund C. Burke, of the Mayo Clinic Department of Pediatrics; Dr. Mark I. Fow, of the Division of Epidemiology and Surveillance, U.S. Public Health Service; Dr. Katherine F. Jeter, of Help for Incontinent People; Dr. Herbert D. Kimmel, of the University of South Florida Department of Psychology; Dr. Edward P. Krenzelok, of the Children's Hospital of Pittsburgh; Dr. F. Mattejat, of the Klinik und Poliklinik fur Kinder- und Jugendpsychiatrie der Philipps-Universitat Marburg; Dr. Robert Prentice, of the American Academy of Pediatrics; Dr. Howard Protinsky, of the Center for Family Services, Virginia Polytechnic Institute and State University; Dr. Edwin W. Reiner; Dr. N. Schmidt, of the Erziehungsberatungsstelle der Stadt Karlsruhe; Dr. Andrew L. Selig; Dr. Larry B. Silver, of the National Institute of Dyslexia; Dr. James M. Stedman, of the University of Texas Medical School at San Antonio; Dr. Gunnar B. Stickler, of the Mayo Clinic Department of Pediatrics; and Dr. W. Thon, of the Akademisches Krankenhaus der Universitat Ulm Department of Urology; and Dr. Harvey A. Tilker supplied valuable information.

Dr. Samuel Himelstein cheerfully offered support. Leah Gorfine and the staff of the Moross Community Center graciously permitted me to use its facilities.

I would like to express my appreciation to Harvey Benovitz, M.D.; Richard Besserman, M.D.; Mr. and Mrs. Nathan Charles; Ray Frenkel; Judy and David K.; the Patashnick family; Carol Topf; Mary Sullivan, of the American Medical Association Division of Library and Information Management, Chicago; Lolita Da Costa and Jane D. Hildreth of the American Psychological Association, Washington; and Michel Konstantyn, of the American Cultural Center Library, Jerusalem.

Finally, and above all, I wish to thank the parents who participated in the development of the Dry All Night method.

Part 1

For Parents

First Aid for Parents

YOU'VE STRUGGLED WITH BEDWETTING LONG ENOUGH. This book is here to help you right now.

This book is designed to help all children who are still wetting at night after they've learned how to read.

That includes

- Girls and boys
- Elementary school and junior high school students (and there are plenty of high school students who still wet!)
- Children who've begun bedwetting after having had a dry period (who, among school-age children, outnumber children who've never been dry)
- Children who wet one or more times a night, one or more times a week, or one or more times a month
- The 10 to 25 percent of bedwetting children who also wet during the daytime (while their day wetting is being treated by a doctor)
- The 10 to 25 percent of bedwetting children who also have difficulty controlling their bowels (while their soiling is being treated by a doctor)
- Children who've been prescribed medication to help their wetting
- Children who live with two parents, with a parent and stepparent, with a single parent, in shared custody, and in any other type of household

Part 1 of this book is for you. It will give you all the information you need to help your child become dry all night. It will explain how you can help your child stop bedwetting as soon as possible, with a minimum of time and effort on your part. And it will help you cope with your child's bedwetting until it stops.

Part 2 of this book is for your child. Research has found that bedwetting stops faster when children take complete responsibility for ending it. Part 2 will make it possible for your child to take that responsibility right now. It

3

consists of a step-by-step method for your child to follow, presented in the form of a picture story.

Before we begin, there are some things you can do starting right now to make things easier on yourself.

First, stop worrying about your child.

Bedwetting isn't an illness. As Dr. Barton D. Schmitt, of the department of pediatrics at the University of Colorado Health Sciences Center, Denver, says, "In a sense, this condition is a normal variation in bladder control rather than a disease state." If bedwetting weren't so bad for a child's self-image, and didn't generate extra laundry, there'd be no need to "do" anything about it. Bedwetting children ranked higher than other children in a test of muscular coordination. A study of more than 1,000 bedwetting children found no difference between their IQs and those of children who didn't wet. One of the world's foremost experts on bedwetting, the eminent British pediatrician Dr. Roy Meadow, once asked a headmaster of an exclusive boarding school whether he accepted bedwetting children. "Certainly," said the headmaster. "They provide most of my scholarship winners!"

And Dr. Meadow makes a point of letting parents know that he wet as a child.

Second, if you've been blaming something you did for your child's wetting, stop right now.

If something a parent did (or didn't do) were capable of causing bedwetting, how could we account for the fact that bedwetting is often hereditary? In a New York University School of Medicine study of doctors' families, 72 percent of children who bedwet had one or two parents who used to wet. Another N.Y.U. study found that children of two parents who bedwet when they were young are more than five times as likely to wet as children whose parents didn't wet. Even children raised apart from their parents have been found to be more likely to bedwet if their parents did.

Your genetic makeup isn't your fault. You were born with it — just as your child was most likely born with a tendency to bedwet.

A good parent isn't necessarily one whose child has no problems at all; that's just a lucky parent. A good parent is one who takes effective action to solve any problems a child may have — and that's what you're going to do, starting right now.

The third thing to do, right this very moment, is give yourself a pat on the back.

Your efforts up till now at dealing with your child's wetting show how much you love your child. A lot of parents haven't had to work as hard as you. All that work is something you can be proud of. The mountain of extra laundry you've had to do is a monument to your dedication as a parent.

4

And above all, you haven't given up hope. Deep down, you know that your child's bedwetting is a parenting challenge that you have the personal resources to meet.

The purpose of the Dry All Night method is to enable you to meet that challenge.

First Aid for Children

As soon as you've absorbed the information in Part 1, you'll be giving this book to your child. Your child is going to be reading Part 2 every day and doing everything it says so he can become dry all night as quickly as possible.

But there are some things you can do right now to help your child become dry all night.

First, if you've been scolding or punishing your child for bedwetting, it's perfectly understandable. After all, you've been through a lot. Only a parent of a child who bedwets can know just how much. But you know it isn't his fault. After all — he does it while he's fast asleep! So effective immediately — stop. Part 2 of this book is going to help your child take complete personal responsibility for becoming dry all night. To take that responsibility, your child is going to need all the support you can give. From now on, the more you cut out every hint of disapproval, the faster bedwetting will cease to be a problem.

Second, starting today, emphasize praise and encouragement in communicating with your child. Just as you know that criticism and negativity from others wouldn't help you learn a new skill, you know that the more you can help your child feel good about himself, the easier it's going to be for him to become dry all night. Every child has his own strengths. Does your child draw well? Is he good in a particular sport? Right now, you can identify some of the areas where your child shines. And beginning today, you can point to his achievements in those areas to let him know just how special you think he is.

Third, up till now, we've been using the term "bedwetting." From now on, let's use a new word:

Sleepwetting.

The real problem, after all, isn't that the bed gets wet. (Step 1 of Part 1 is going to tell you how to solve that problem immediately.)

The real problem is that your child wets while he's sleeping.

The issue, in other words, isn't what your child wets. It's when your child wets!

"Bedwetting" is a word that has, unintentionally, done a lot of harm. By dwelling on that soggy piece of furniture, it has caused generations of parents to get angry at their kids. It has made parents forget that their children are a lot more valuable and delicate than their home furnishings. And it has filled children with guilt about the damage it suggests that they're doing.

A wet mattress can be aired out. Smelly bedding can be thrown in the washing machine. The hurt felt by a child who has been repeatedly yelled at or smacked for behavior over which he has no control doesn't go away so easily.

Not to mention the likelihood that the stress a child experiences when a parent hits the ceiling because of a wet bed can, ironically, prolong the problem.

So from now on — let's say "sleepwetting": the more we spread the word, the sooner "bedwetting" will fade away.

And let's not substitute "sleepwetter" for "bedwetter." From now on, let's just say, "a child who sleepwets." Would we call a child who has hay fever "a sneezer"? We'd never use a word that might suggest that sneezing represented a child's identity.

It's always a bad idea to hang labels on people describing what they do when what we want is for them to stop doing it. Labels imply permanency; the Dry All Night method is about change. By using terms that don't label, you'll be telling your child that change is possible.

You may want to come up with a special positive way of referring to your child. It stands to reason that a child who's referred to as "my little ballerina" or "my assistant chef" or "my champion gymnast" or "my junior quarterback" is going to become dry all night a lot faster than one who's been labeled negatively.

How This Book Came to Be

SOON AFTER THE PUBLICATION of my book for getting toddlers out of diapers, *Toilet Learning: The Picture Book Technique for Children and Parents,* I began receiving letters from parents of school-age children, like this one from a mother in Maspeth, New York:

> I am also asking for my girlfriend as she has her son who is seven years old and he bedwets every night. She keeps him in diapers every night and still has him sleeping in a crib, still waiting for him to stop his bedwetting so she can get him a bed. Can you offer her any advice as to the bedwetting or a book she can get? Also, do you think he's too old to be in diapers at night and sleeping in a crib?

Between the lines of those letters (which often asked for help for "a friend"), I could feel the hurt of both children and parents. Imagine being seven years old — a second-grader, able to read and write and add and subtract — still in diapers, still sleeping in a crib! I wrote back immediately to everyone who sent me letters like that, reassuring them, giving advice. But there was no book I could recommend. And there might never be one.

Unless I wrote it myself . . .

As time went by, more and more parents asked me to write a book designed to stop sleepwetting. "Why don't you do it the same way you did *Toilet Learning*?" they said. "You could combine a section for parents with a picture book for children showing the things they should do."

A few parents wondered whether it was really necessary to do anything about sleepwetting. "Kids grow out of it sooner or later, don't they?" they asked.

I obtained reports of research on that question and found that "grow out of it" they do — at the rate of about 14 percent a year. In other words, if nothing is done, 1 out of 7 children who wet becomes dry each year.

But that meant the chances were 6 out of 7 that any given child who sleepwet would still be wetting a year later!

Unless something was done for them, 74 percent of children who sleepwet would still be wetting two years later, 64 percent three years later, and 55 percent four years later. When I thought of the cost of sleepwetting — to children's feelings about themselves, to family harmony — I found these odds far too high.

As I thought more about it, a book-based method for stopping sleep-wetting seemed like a good idea, for several reasons.

First, putting a book in a child's hands places the responsibility for stopping sleepwetting where a landmark University of California study has shown it's most effective: with the child. And, of course, giving the child full responsibility for becoming dry means less work for parents (and less chance of conflict with the child that will result in stress that can cause sleepwetting to continue).

Second, the age at which children become capable of taking responsibility for stopping sleepwetting just happens to be around the age when they learn to read. So a book designed to stop sleepwetting can be used by parents to tell if their child is ready to take charge. If the child is old enough to read and understand the picture story (with assistance from parents in the beginning, if necessary), the child is old enough to follow the steps for becoming dry all night that are described in the story on her own.

Third, a picture book makes it possible for children who sleepwet to use a technique known in behavioral pediatrics as "peer modeling." The child is reassured and encouraged by seeing other children doing things to become dry all night.

Fourth, a picture book designed to stop sleepwetting brings into play one of the most important educational principles — repetition. Many parents had written to tell me that *Toilet Learning* was their children's favorite book and that they had read it over and over again. So I knew that children would repeatedly read a book about controlling their own bodies.

Fifth, a child who sleepwets often feels as if she's the only one in the whole world, and that there's nothing she can do about it. Giving this book to your child will say to her, "There are enough kids who wet for there to be a whole book about it. And there's plenty you can do!" Once children who wet begin to realize that they aren't alone and that they do have the power to control their bodies, they're already well on their way to becoming dry.

So I decided to develop a book-based method that would do the job. The volume you hold in your hands is the result.

A last word before you begin the Dry All Night method.

A baby horse is able to stand right after it's born — and its parents don't have to help with its first steps. We humans need a little more parental assistance to get us on our feet. But we have a similar inborn impulse toward being able to function in an adult manner. The tiniest baby will step left-right-left-right-left if held up by the hands and gently "walked" along so that its feet touch a flat surface. You were able to teach your child to walk only because she already possessed an inborn need, desire, ability, and tendency to stand on her own two feet.

I believe that every child has a deep inner need, desire, ability, and tendency to be dry all night. Becoming dry is a natural part of every child's striving for mastery and autonomy. Our job as parents is simply to remove the obstacles, and point the way.

Perhaps you feel you've been laboring under a special burden. May I suggest that you've been provided with a special gift? This is a precious time for you and your child — a time of being together that you'll never have again. Many parents who never had your "problem" wake up one day and realize that their children are no longer young, that with all the distractions of daily coping they never really had a chance to concentrate on guiding their development the way they would have liked to. Consider yourself fortunate that necessity is giving you an unparalleled opportunity to focus on your child's needs.

Being the parent of a child who sleepwets is certainly a challenge. But having been able to help a child stop sleepwetting is a privilege. Long after the inconvenience of your child's wetting is a dim memory, the knowledge that you used the process of helping your child to become dry all night as a way of becoming closer will remain as a proud possession.

It is my hope that you will find this book as rewarding to use as I found it to write.

10 Steps That Will Help Your Child Become Dry All Night

Before familiarizing yourself with these ten steps for helping your child become dry all night, I suggest that you breeze through Part 2 of this book once, to get an overall feel for what we're going to have your child doing — and then return to

Step 1: Lighten Your Sleepwetting Load

There is always a best way of doing everything . . .

— Emerson

YOU MAY FEEL that you're at your wits' end, coping with soggy, smelly laundry. You need relief — and this section is going to give it to you.

Some children who follow the Dry All Night method will stop sleepwetting literally overnight. Others will take days, still others could take weeks. Some might even take months. For you to help your child become dry by eliminating as much stress as possible from his life, it's important for you to be relaxed and cheerful, regardless of how long your child needs to develop at his own pace. And soaked bedding can throw a wet blanket over your entire day.

Of course, you want your child to stop sleepwetting primarily for his sake, not yours. But so that you'll be better able to help him, give yourself the gift of minimizing your involvement with wet bedding. The less energy you need to put into running a laundry service, the more energy you'll have for your crucial role of providing support and encouragement to your child.

UNDERPADS AND DRAWSHEETS

The key to parental survival of sleepwetting is to use special "underpads" or "drawsheets" to keep the bed from getting wet in the first place.

Disposable underpads are used in hospitals and by incontinent adults to protect bedding. Known in the trade as "blue pads," they're made of moisture-absorbing cellulose fiber bonded to a plastic backing. Such brands as Depend and Curity are available in supermarkets and drugstores, along with stores' own brands. Montgomery Ward, J. C. Penney, and Sears carry their own brands. Various sizes are available. Those that are best for sleep-wetting have one dimension of about 36 inches, so that they can cover the entire width of the bed.

One brand of underpad I particularly recommend is Tuckables. Tuckables solve the slippage problem by being what they sound like — tuckable. The plastic backing extends 17 inches beyond each side of the absorbent pad, creating "wings" to be tucked underneath the mattress on both sides of the bed. And Tuckables are available with absorbent pads up to 36 inches square — big enough to accommodate even a child who moves up and down the bed a great deal while sleeping. You can get information on where to find Tuckables in your area by contacting the manufacturer:

Hosposables Products, Inc.
P.O. Box 387
Central Jersey Industrial Park
Bound Brook, NJ 08805
Fax: (201)469-0769
Telephone: (201)469-8700
Toll-Free: 1-800-221-1302

Another good brand of disposable underpads is Dri-Sheet. The plastic backing of Dri-Sheet 30-inch-square pads has adhesive strips to attach the underpad to the sheet so that it won't slide around. For information on where to obtain Dri-Sheet underpads in your area, you can contact the manufacturer:

Paper-Pak Products, Inc.
1941 White Ave.
P.O. Box 1060
La Verne, CA 91750
Telephone: (714)392-1200
Toll-Free: 1-800-635-4560

Disposable underpads make life with sleepwetting a lot easier, but they can be fairly expensive. If you can afford the temporary cost, I urge you to use them, because they're the easiest way of cutting down on making beds and doing laundry. You'll be better able to help your child if you let your pocketbook absorb the wear and tear, rather than your nervous system.

If the cost of disposable underpads is a serious problem, you can use a washable absorbent drawsheet to cover the midsection of the bed. Drawsheets have a waterproof backing and go across the bed, tucking under the mattress on both sides. (Tuckables could be described as disposable drawsheets.) Drawsheets are available at sickroom supplies departments of drug stores. I like the Style 102 "3-in-1" MED-I-PAD Incontinence Draw. One of these costs about as much as 20 throwaway Tuckables, but it can be laundered many times. You can obtain information on where to find the Style 102 drawsheet from the manufacturer:

> MED-I-PANT Inc.
> 4100 Parthais
> Montreal, Que. H2K 3T9
> Canada
> Fax: (514)522-8448
> Telephone: (514)522-1224
> U.S. Toll-Free: 1-800-361-4964

In the past it was sometimes suggested that children be required to strip the bed and change sheets and blankets in the middle of the night or in the morning, in the belief that children should deal with what the late child psychologist Rudolf Dreikurs called the "natural and logical consequences" of their actions. Dr. Dreikurs, however, meant that children ought to be the ones to wash off walls they've scribbled on — not that they should have to struggle with unwieldy sheets and blankets because of muscular contractions that happen without their knowledge and against their will. Because changing sheets and blankets is difficult for children, it's likely to be perceived by them as a form of punishment. And punishment results in stress that can prolong sleepwetting.

Fortunately, children usually don't find it hard to change wet underpads or drawsheets. So they can experience the sense of maturity that comes from coping with their wetting without feeling that they're being punished. So if you use underpads, keep a supply in a place in your child's room where he can reach them easily. Show him where to throw away the wet underpad if he is awakened by an "accident," and how to put a fresh one on the bed. A plastic garbage pail with a lid, kept in the child's room just for underpads, lined with a garbage bag and rinsed out regularly, will help control odor. If you prefer reusable drawsheets, keep several in his room, and show him where to put them if they get wet.

If your child doesn't like to change underpads or drawsheets, don't make an issue out of it. Any positive effect from changing them depends on the child's wanting to do it. Forcing a child won't help.

LIFTING

Have you been "lifting" your child — waking him up before he sleepwets, or taking him to the bathroom to urinate while he's sleeping?

If so, I congratulate you. You've taken the initiative. You've been doing something to try to help your child.

I sympathize with you. As a working mother of four, I know how hard it is to keep ahead of kids' laundry!

I congratulate you for it — I sympathize with you for it — but I'd like you to stop.

Surveys by the Ambulatory Pediatric Association have found that lifting was the most common response to sleepwetting. Between 67 and 84 percent of parents said they lifted their children.

But there's no evidence that lifting can "train" a child to be dry. Scientific reports do not indicate that lifting helps. The authors of a University of Toronto study said that lifting of children attending their sleepwetting clinic "probably delayed a cure." And another study found that children whose treatment included lifting improved more slowly than those who weren't lifted.

Lifting can make a child feel that only others can control his sleepwetting. And it can create tensions that will interfere with becoming dry. As Dr. Alan D. Perlmutter, chief of pediatric urology at Children's Hospital of Michigan, Detroit, has said, "In many cases, the effort and discipline of frequent awakening stimulate latent or overt hostility in the parents, and anger or anxiety in the child." Most children — not just those who sleepwet — are pretty hard to wake up in the middle of the night. It's never a good idea to set parents and children up for an unnecessary battle of wills, especially one scheduled for a time when both are tired.

In the past, lifting was the only way a parent could keep the bed from getting soaked. But modern technology now makes it possible to keep the bed dry with less effort — and without disturbing children's sleep.

So if you're lifting your child, it's time to stop, because it isn't really helping. If it were, you wouldn't be reading this book!

SHEETS AND BLANKETS

Ideally, children who sleepwet should have knitted or knitted terry sheets that don't require ironing or folding. So that the bed can be made as easily as possible, the bottom sheets should be fitted at all four corners. The top sheet, which will help keep the (washable!) blanket dry, should be fitted at the foot end. A good brand of knitted sheets — 100 percent cotton, fitted top and bottom with no elastic to wear out — is Sleep-Knit, manufactured by

> Sleep-Knit International
> P.O. Box 4698
> 67 Holly Hill Lane
> Greenwich, CT 06830
> Fax: (203)869-1671
> Telephone: (203)869-4336

If sheets or blankets get wet, you should be the one to change them unless your child is old enough, big enough, and strong enough to do it easily, and actively wants to.

Airing sheets and blankets outdoors can remove odor from them without washing. From a health standpoint, there's no need to wash them, since normal urine contains no bacteria. To control odor, wet sheets, blankets, and pajamas waiting to be laundered should either be placed in the washing machine immediately, or kept in an airtight hamper.

MATTRESSES AND PILLOWS

One approach that helps peace of mind is to use an inexpensive foam mattress — better, to have two, so that if one gets wet and has to be aired out, you'll have a spare.

Especially if you use a more expensive mattress, it should be covered with plastic or rubber. Cheap or improvised mattress covers that leak, crack, or tear can let you down. You can buy a heavy-duty, hospital-strength cover that encases the mattress on the top, bottom, and sides from drugstore sickroom supplies departments. Pillow covers are also available. I recommend the following top-quality models, available by mail from

> United Linen Inc.
> P.O. Box 508
> 1252 Brunswick Ave.
> Far Rockaway, NY 11691
> Telephone: (718)337-6600

No. MC3975VZ1 Bed Protector — Vinyl — 39" × 75" — for twin bed
No. MC2127VZ1 Bed Protector — Vinyl — 21" × 27" — for pillow

PAJAMAS

Several pairs of pajamas should always be available in your child's room for him to change into if he is awakened by an "accident." This means owning a bunch of extra pajamas so that there's no rush about washing them. Show him where you want him to put wet pajamas.

If the weather is warm enough, or the temperature inside the house is set high enough, your child can sleep without bottoms (or tops, too) to lower the laundry level.

DIAPERS

I've known parents who kept their children in diapers at night as late as seven, eight, nine, even twelve years of age. But wearing diapers makes a child feel like a baby, and feeling like a baby only prolongs sleepwetting. Not to mention the fact that a child who is wearing a diaper is going to have a hard time urinating in the toilet in the middle of the night. No child who's old enough to read this book should be wearing diapers to bed, even if he wets every single night. And children who've been taken out of diapers should never be threatened with being put back into them.

It's true that it takes a bit of creativity for parents to cope with the effects of sleepwetting without using diapers. But it's a lot easier than coping with the negative effects on a school-age child of still being in diapers.

If your child has been wearing diapers to sleep, first use the information in this step to help you protect his bedding while he's becoming dry all night. Once you've got your "bedding protection system" in place, tell him, "Now that you're getting so big and grown-up, you don't need to wear diapers anymore."

Even children who also wet during the day shouldn't wear diapers. Diapers are a symbol of babyishness, and you want to do everything possible to emphasize that your child is becoming a "big kid" who is soon going to be urinating only in the toilet. Instead of diapers, use disposable absorbent contoured inserts, also known as shields. They're made of the same material as disposable diapers — fiber pad on the inside, plastic cover on the outside. But since they're designed to be worn by incontinent adults, they don't imply that the person wearing them is babyish.

Contoured absorbent inserts will fit inside a child's knitted brief or panty. Because of the thickness of the insert, you may want your child to wear a larger size of outer pants so that he'll be able to move freely and so that the bulk won't show from the outside. He can keep a supply of inserts in his backpack or locker and change them as needed, using a toilet stall for privacy. Place each fresh insert in a separate opaque bag, such as the brown paper lunch bags that can be found in supermarkets, usually shelved near sandwich bags, freezer bags, and food storage bags. The bag will prevent other children from seeing the insert, embarrassing your child, and he can put the wet insert he has just taken off into it before throwing it in the garbage. Make sure your child understands that used inserts can't be flushed down the toilet.

Such brands as Attends, Depend Shields, and Surety Shields are available in supermarkets and drugstores. Sears carries its own brand. Depend Shields have three adhesive tabs that attach to underwear to prevent them from slipping around. Serenity shields are contoured especially for women and are good for girls. Surety Shields have an adhesive strip and the advantage of containing a deodorant. MaxiShield Shaped Inserts have an adhesive strip and elastic gathers around the legs to prevent leakage, but no deodorant. You can obtain information on who carries MaxiShield in your area from the manufacturer:

> Whitestone Products
> 40 Turner Place
> Piscataway, NJ 08854
> Telephone: (201)752-2700
> Toll-Free: 1-800-526-3567

Contoured inserts come in several absorbencies. If you find that the highest-absorbency inserts don't hold your child's urine output, and if your child is large enough, you can use an adult-incontinence product known as "undergarments." Undergarments come up higher in the front and back and hold more liquid. Depend Undergarments, a popular brand, have elastic gathers around the legs and are held in place by reusable elastic straps supplied in the package.

You can direct-order inserts and undergarments by the case from

> Home Delivery Incontinent Supplies Co. (HDIS)
> P.O. Box 3465
> St. Louis, MO 63143
> In Missouri or Canada: (314)389-4134
> Toll-Free: 1-800-538-1036

If your child has been wetting during the day, explain to him that he can help himself to become dry all day by urinating at specific times, approximately every two hours during the daytime, according to a list the child can make himself, carry with him, and check off. The exact times should be chosen to fall, to the extent possible, during recesses, class breaks, and lunch. Tell your child's teachers that he has difficulty controlling urination during the daytime. Explain to them the importance of regular urinations — and ask them never to embarrass your child by public reminders (let alone teasing!) Don't tell them that your child sleepwets — let that be a secret between you and your child.

SKIN PROTECTION

If your child's skin becomes irritated by urine, you can protect it with a layer of petroleum jelly, such as Vaseline or generic petrolatum U.S.P. Numerous "barrier film" products, such as Depend Barrier Cream, designed for incontinent adults, are available as aerosols, creams, and wipes in sickroom supply departments. They tend to be rather expensive, and most are just glorified petroleum jelly. But you may find that one of them is more suitable for your child's skin.

ROOM DEODORIZERS

Many parents have told me that one of the things they find most bothersome about sleepwetting is the smell of urine. But I've found that often they weren't doing anything specific about controlling odor. Even if you've gotten used to the smell, it's bound to give you a lift to put room deodorizers wherever they'll improve the atmosphere — in your child's room, in the laundry room — and to use a spray air freshener frequently.

PARENTS WITH SEPARATE HOUSEHOLDS

If your child will be spending the night in another household regularly, discuss this step of Part 1 with the noncustodial or shared-custody parent (or other adult), and make sure that the other household has a supply of items you're using, such as absorbent inserts, fitted sheets, bed- and pillow-protectors, underpads, drawsheets, and barrier film.

ALARMS

Electronic alarms that sound when the child wets became popular in England in the 1950s but haven't been received well here. Of 446 doctors in a recent Ambulatory Pediatric Association survey, 15 said they usually suggested it. "Perhaps one of the reasons this method has never become popular in this country," says Dr. Larry McLain of the pediatrics department of the University of Illinois College of Medicine, "is that physicians feel the conditioning treatment may be psychologically harmful to the child." In my experience, the most common problem with the alarm is that instead of the child waking up when it sounds, the parent does. As a result, parents stop using it. They don't want to try solving a problem that's driving them crazy by using an approach that drives them crazier.

If you've been able to live with the alarm, there's no need to discontinue it before starting to use this book. This book is designed to help your child learn to wake up before he wets or to sleep through the night without wetting. As either begins to happen, the alarm will stop sounding. When your child stops sleepwetting, he can stop both using the alarm and reading Part 2.

Step 2: Realize That Sleepwetting Is a Common Problem

Nothing is fair or good alone.

— Emerson

DID YOU EVER FEEL that you were all alone with your child's sleepwetting? As if you were the only parent in the world with such a problem? Well, you're not.

If you've felt alone, it was because of the wall of silence that surrounds sleepwetting.

We live in a talkative society. We've got talk shows, morning, noon, and night. We've got happy-talk on the local TV news. We've got 24-hour call-in radio. We've got hot lines. We've got chat lines. We've got CB in our pickups. We've got cellular phones in our cars. We've got teleconferencing in our offices. Call Waiting says there's a call waiting.

And people talk about everything.

People talk about alcoholism.

People talk about drug addiction.

People talk about talk-show hosts.

There's nothing people don't talk about.

Except sleepwetting.

I know a public relations executive who has two children who sleep-wet — a girl, thirteen, and a boy, five. "Only I, my husband, my kids, and my doctor know about it," she told me. "My mother doesn't know. Neither does my father. I've never told any of my other relatives. My friends don't know. My neighbors don't know. Nobody at work knows."

This woman isn't the quiet type. Her profession is communication. Yet for her, as for most parents, sleepwetting is the Child-Rearing Problem That Dare Not Speak Its Name.

Much of this silence is a good thing, because it protects children from embarrassment. In fact, I tell parents that the fewer people who know that their child sleepwets, the faster she'll become dry all night. But the fact that sleepwetting is one of the great untalked-about topics of our time has one extremely damaging side effect: it makes sleepwetting an unheard-of phenomenon.

The wall of silence around sleepwetting creates the illusion that children who wet at night are few and far between. It fosters the impression that the parents of such children suffer from a rare and curious affliction. Yet the truth is that sleepwetting is one of the most common ongoing childhood conditions — if not the most common.

A massive study, tracking the development of 4,294 children born during the same week, found that more than 10 percent were sleepwetting at age six and that over 5 percent were wetting when they were eleven. The landmark study conducted by the research team of Sears, Maccoby, and Levin, found that 19 percent of children aged five to six wet while they were sleeping. A survey of Texas children aged six to ten found that 21 percent wet at night. In a survey by researchers at Johns Hopkins University, Baltimore, 20 percent of children between the ages of six and thirteen were found to sleepwet at least once a week. In another survey, 16 percent of ten-year-olds were found to be wetting at night.

The Ambulatory Pediatric Association recently conducted a survey of parents of 1,379 children in New York, Pennsylvania, Nebraska, Minnesota, Missouri, Ohio, and New Hampshire. It found that 25 percent of children aged six through eleven were sleepwetting, with 13 percent of twelve- to eighteen-year-olds still not dry at night.

Surprised at how big these numbers are? Yet sleepwetting may really be even more common.

When I set out to find parents to work with me in developing the Dry All Night method, I thought I was going to have a hard time finding families with children who sleepwet. But it turned out that just about every parent I spoke to either had a child who sleepwet or knew one that did. Among large families, the percentage that had at least one child who sleepwet approached 100. I was left with the feeling that there may be a fair amount of "closet sleepwetting" out there that researchers have no way of picking up on. Because there are undoubtedly parents who, when asked by a stranger whether their child does something people don't want to talk about, don't want to talk about it.

So it's time to subtract loneliness from the difficulties you've been coping with. There are millions of you out there!

A child who wets at night often thinks she's the only person in the whole wide world who has this problem. After all, she has never seen any children sleepwet on TV. She has probably never heard any of her friends or classmates say they sleepwet. As a result, she may feel there's something "wrong" with her. Feeling like that isn't going to help her become dry all night.

Now that you realize that you're not alone, it's important for your child to be reassured that she's not alone. Part 2 of this book will be driving this point home to your child every day. And here's an easy-to-remember fact that will help you reassure her:

A recent study found that among eleven-year-olds the proportion who sleepwet is — 11 percent.

When you emphasize to your child that even among the eleven-year-olds she knows, 1 out of every 9 may sleepwet, it'll be clear to her that there's nothing "babyish" about sleepwetting. She'll realize that children of all ages wet while they're sleeping.

They just don't talk about it.

Step 3: Confront Your Feelings about Sleepwetting

To different minds, the same world is a hell, and a heaven.

— Emerson

HAVE YOU BEEN DOING any of these things?

- Teasing a child about sleepwetting
- Criticizing a child for sleepwetting
- Comparing a sleepwetting child with other children
- Expressing hopelessness about sleepwetting
- Name-calling for having sleepwet
- Threatening to punish a child for sleepwetting
- Punishing a child for having sleepwet
- Spanking a child for having sleepwet
- Expressing rejection of a child for sleepwetting
- Shaming a child in front of others for sleepwetting

If so, it's perfectly understandable. After all, you've been through a lot. Only a parent of a child who sleepwets can know just how much. But it's important to phase out any negativity you've inadvertently been putting out.

Any stress your child experiences can prolong sleepwetting. Stress can even trigger sleepwetting in children who've previously been dry. And any negativity a parent conveys to a child is going to cause stress.

We parents aren't machines, and there's no switch we can throw to turn off the negativity. Counting to ten and breathing deeply are better than ex-

21

ploding but aren't the answer. Children who sleepwet tend to be especially sensitive, and negativity that's under control will be perceived by them as exactly that: negativity that's under control. If we try to just bottle up our anger, sooner or later the cork is going to pop. The really effective way to stop projecting negative feelings about sleepwetting is — to stop having them.

Dr. Thomas Phaer's 1544 *Boke of Children,* the first treatise on pediatrics in the English language, featured a section entitled

OF PYSSYING IN THE BEDDE

Many times for debility of vertus retentive of the reines or blader, as wel olde men as children are oftentimes annoyed, whan their urine issueth out either in theyre slepe or waking against theyr wylles, having no power to reteine it whan it cometh, therefore yf they will be holpen, fyrst they must avoid al fat meates, til ye vertue be restored againe, and to use this pouder in their meates and drynkes.

Take the wesand [windpipe] of a cocke, and plucke it, then brenne it in pouder, and use of it twise or thryes a daye. The stones of an hedge-hogge poudred is of the same vertue.

If powdered rooster windpipe didn't help much, at least it didn't hurt. But it wasn't long before sleepwetting was being treated with supposedly more advanced methods. In 1612 the prominent Paris physician Jacques Guille-meau recommended threatening and shaming as cures for sleepwetting.

By the nineteenth century, doctors had soured on this kind of harshness. Dr. Samuel Adams, writing about sleepwetting in the *American Journal of Obstetrics* in 1844, was critical of certain of his colleagues: "Simply because some are not able, by a careless and superficial examination to find the cause, and well knowing that their reputations will be at stake if they do not account for the act, they too often condemn the helpless child to daily flog-gings."

Today, we know that threatening, shaming, or hitting a child who sleep-wets can only prolong the problem. One of the most important principles in educational psychology is called the Yerkes-Dobson law. It says that anxiety interferes with learning. This applies to any educational process, from learning the letters of the alphabet to learning to pilot a supersonic jet.

And how do you suppose the Yerkes-Dobson law was originally formulated, back in 1908? In the course of conducting research on sleepwetting!

Becoming dry all night involves a learning process, so stress interferes with it. A University of Wisconsin study has found that "night training was retarded by the use of negative interpersonal reinforcement" (such as scolding, spanking, criticism, and name-calling) and "negative external reinforcement" (for example, refusing to change wet pajamas).

In addition to interfering with becoming dry, stress can cause sleepwetting to start after a child has been dry — what is known in scientific terminology as "secondary enuresis" or "onset enuresis." Dr. John S. Werry, of the University of New Zealand School of Medicine, one of the world's foremost authorities on sleepwetting, has written, "In my own series of 58 cases of onset enuresis (reappearance after a period of continence), the overwhelmingly commonest cause could be seen to be environmental variables likely to provoke a high level of anxiety in the child." In another study, researchers actually recorded increased pressure inside the bladder when stress-producing topics were discussed.

The reason parents express negative feelings toward children who sleepwet is that they have negative ideas about sleepwetting. But I've found that when parents take a hard look at those ideas, they realize they don't make sense, and change them. From then on, they discover that they have no more negative feelings to express.

Some of the most common ideas parents tell me they have about sleepwetting go like this:

- "It doesn't bother him. He doesn't mind lying in it. He couldn't care less about stopping."
- "He does it on purpose. It's his way of getting attention. He's trying to get back at me."
- "All this laundry's killing me. The smell drives me up the wall. I can't take it anymore."

I've never known a child who sleepwet who wasn't bothered by it. Nobody enjoys sleeping in a puddle. But like everyone else, children sometimes hide their inner pain. The chances are that your child wants to be dry even more than you want him to be.

One mother told me that her six-year-old wet because he wanted attention. I asked her how she knew. She replied that recently he'd been in the hospital for a hernia operation. Before, he'd been wetting every night. While in the hospital, he was dry. When he came home, she gave him lots of attention — asking him how he felt, playing games with him, reading to him. While he was recovering, he didn't wet once. When he went back to school, he began wetting again.

I explained that it's common for children to stop sleepwetting while they're away from home. It's likely that the wetting ceases because their sleep, disturbed by being in a strange place, is lighter. After several nights, they may get used to their new surroundings and sleep more deeply, so that the wetting starts again.

The fact that this mother's child was dry when he was receiving a great deal of attention didn't show that his wetting when he wasn't receiving it was deliberate — it simply showed that giving him attention helped his wetting (as, in my experience, it usually does). If someone's heart is racing because he's afraid, and you give him attention and his heart slows down, you don't conclude that he made his heart beat quickly on purpose. And you certainly wouldn't conclude that the person's increased heart rate was something he was doing to you!

As Dr. Roger Broughton, professor of neurology at the University of Ottawa School of Medicine, one of the world's top experts on children's sleep disorders, says, "The concept that bedwetting is semivoluntary or a voluntary aggressive activity can definitely be abandoned."

When parents say, "The smell drives me up the wall," they actually mean, "I don't like the odor of urine." "All this laundry's killing me," really means, "All this laundry irritates me." It's natural for us to exaggerate a little — as long as we don't believe our exaggerations. Following Step 2 will help you minimize the laundry and control the odor. But in general, if we feel we have to let off steam, it's easier on our nerves to replace overstatements like "I can't take it anymore" with low-key expressions such as, "I sure do wish this would stop."

If you have strong negative feelings about sleepwetting, chances are that when you analyze your ideas carefully, your negativity will fade away. But if you continue to feel some anger about sleepwetting, it's important to lengthen your fuse.

The thing to do with any anger that remains is to let it out — but not on your child. You can talk about your anger with a close friend or a professional. The same goes if you're feeling depressed. If sleepwetting has got you down, you need someone to cheer you up. The ideal person to ventilate to is another parent with a child who sleepwets. It's best not to talk to a relative who has contact with your child, so as to minimize the number of people around your child who know about his wetting.

Sleepwetting is so common that it shouldn't take too many phone calls to find a friend who'll be surprised and relieved to find that someone else has the same problem. Large families are particularly likely to include a child who wets.

If you feel embarrassed by calling your existing friends, I recommend looking for a new one or two. You can put up notices on bulletin boards with just your telephone number. Or you can even run a classified ad in the newspaper, or in a shopper or pennysaver, announcing, "Parent of sleepwetter wishes to share experiences with other parents who have same problem."

You can talk out your frustration one-on-one. Or, if you locate several parents, you can organize an informal support group that will meet every so often to share feelings and experiences. If you should find yourself reaching your boiling point, you can prevent any anger from spilling over onto your child by putting in an emergency call to a parent with the same problem — your own personal sleepwetting "hot line."

While I'm on the subject of expressing one's feelings, keep in mind that negativity is what we respond with when something's blocking our path. Feelings of negativity melt away when we're making progress in a self-fulfilling activity. Your child is going to be taking personal responsibility for becoming dry all night. With this problem largely off your hands, what better time to develop ways of expressing yourself? If the smell of wet bedding has you down, mix perfumes using essential oils or plant an herb garden to pamper your nose. If running a laundry service hasn't been your idea of a creative outlet, tie-dye fabrics, or make batiks. If you're tired of thinking about toilets, do your own ceramics. Dance. Weave. Paint. Refinish antiques. Weld found objects together and call it sculpture. Make wine at home.

And if all else fails, take up acting. Maybe you won't be able to get rid of all your negativity. If so, when you're around your child, instead of being the real frazzled you, act the part of an expert nanny you've hired to take charge — relaxed, cheerful, confident, amply compensated, with a month of paid vacation and Thursdays off. Transform yourself into an elderly teacher, wise, experienced, the type younger teachers come to for advice. Or make believe you're a parenting educator showing an audience of had-it-up-to-here parents how to keep cool under pressure. If you've ever been onstage, you know that there comes a point when you begin to live the emotions you're portraying.

If despite all your efforts you feel that you're about to express negative feelings to your child, minimize the stress that results by making a statement about yourself, rather than about your child: "It annoys me so much when you sleepwet." And rather than yelling at a child, a parent can quietly say, "When you sleepwet, it makes me so angry I feel like screaming."

TEASING

It's natural to feel like poking a bit of fun at a child for sleepwetting. It releases tension. It shows that you can manage a smile about the problem. But children tend to be quite sensitive about their sleepwetting. Teasing them about it can hurt their feelings, even if they grin and bear it. And it can cause stress that will make the problem continue. So don't tease. And see to it that your child's brothers, sisters, and relatives don't make fun of your child for sleepwetting — or for anything else.

CRITICIZING

The most patient parent may sometimes feel like criticizing a child for sleep-wetting. But criticizing is counterproductive. Even nonverbal criticism — a tsk, a sigh, a groan, a gesture, a roll of the eyes — will produce stress that can result in more sleepwetting. And like any form of negativity, a child's fear that there will be more of it in the future can cause additional stress. Children tend to believe what adults say to them. Telling a child, "You can't do anything right!" is likely to be a self-fulfilling prophecy. There's no down-side risk in saying, "Come on — you can do it!"

COMPARING

It's understandable to have the impulse to compare a sleepwetting child to other children. But it doesn't help to say things like, "Why can't you be dry like so-and-so?" or even, "Why can't you read Part 2 and do everything it says like so-and-so?" Comparisons tend to make children feel inadequate. Becoming dry all night isn't a race. Children should be measured by the extent to which they're fulfilling their own potential, not according to how they stack up to others.

EXPRESSING HOPELESSNESS

It can be frustrating to be the parent of a child who sleepwets, and it's normal to feel like saying, "You'll never be dry!" Expressing hopelessness about sleepwetting may reflect a parent's fear that if dryness isn't attained at the expected age, it may never be attained. But this fear isn't justified by the facts. Sooner or later, children stop; the purpose of this book is simply to help them stop sooner, rather than later.

The late psychologist Dr. O. H. Mowrer pointed out that hope for positive reinforcement is an indispensable motivation for learning. The main positive reinforcement a child should hope to receive for following the Dry All Night method should be — to become dry all night. If a parent tells the child he'll never be dry, the parent is only saying it to let off steam, but the child has no way of knowing that the parent doesn't believe it. To a child's ears, such statements chip away at hope for dryness. And if there's no hope for dryness, why should the child read Part 2 and follow its steps?

NAME-CALLING

Parents call children names with the intention of helping them, by getting them to change. But calling a child a name for having sleepwet doesn't help, because children tend to live up to the expectations they hear expressed by their parents. Call a child a brat and he'll be one.

THREATENING

Sometimes threats have a way of sneaking in when we don't even mean them. A parent may say to a child who wakes up after a wet night, "You shower and get that smell off you before you go to school or I'll brain you." It's easier on both parent and child if a nonthreatening approach is used, assuming cooperation rather than demanding it: "I bet the smell of urine bothers you. I think you'll feel a lot more comfortable after you take a nice hot shower."

When a parent threatens to punish a child for sleepwetting, it's an attempt to buy time. The parent doesn't really want to punish the child, so instead lets the child off with a warning. But if a parent threatens to punish and then doesn't make good on the threat, the child first experiences stress and then is relieved to learn that things the parent says don't have to be taken seriously. If a parent threatens to punish and then does punish, the child first experiences stress — and then experiences worse stress.

PUNISHING

Punishing a child can be an expression of love. But punishments don't have to be harsh to be effective. When a child deliberately misbehaves, the disapproval expressed by a calm, firm, "I don't like what you just did, and I don't want you to do it anymore" can sometimes be the most effective punishment. But punishing a child in any way for sleepwetting won't help. A child can't be held accountable for things his body does while he's out cold. And punishment will create stress that can only prolong the problem.

Not only intentional punishment should be avoided, but anything the child might interpret as punishment. For instance, the seven-year-old I mentioned earlier who was still in a crib at age seven wasn't being kept there as a deliberate punishment — his mother was "still waiting for him to stop his bedwetting so she can get him a bed." But I would bet that the child experienced sleeping in a crib, when all his friends had long been sleeping in beds, as a severe punishment.

SPANKING

It's best to save spanking for serious, intentional misbehavior. Sleepwetting isn't misbehavior at all, so spanking for it only makes a child feel misunderstood. In fact, spanking for any reason can be so stressful to a child that it can actually trigger a sleepwetting incident.

EXPRESSING REJECTION

I know that parents don't mean it when they say, "I hate you when you sleepwet" — they know they don't mean it — but their children don't know they don't mean it. Besides, a parent wouldn't say, "I can't stand you when you yawn." A child who likes himself is going to become dry all night sooner. You can help your child like himself all the time by making sure he knows that you like him all the time — while keeping to yourself any dislike you may have for his sleepwetting.

SHAMING

It's normal to want to talk about something that's bothering you. But telling someone that a child sleepwets when the child is present can make the child feel ashamed. Even if the child isn't there when somebody else is told, the child can be embarrassed if the other person later mentions his sleepwetting in his presence. The safest rule is for parents never to talk about a child's sleepwetting to their own friends (unless, as recommended previously, for needed ventilation, or for experience-sharing with parents of children who sleepwet), the child's friends, or relatives, even if the child isn't there.

We all slip up once in a while. If you inadvertently do one of the above things, explanation and reassurance from you will help reduce stress. You can say something like this: "You know, when you sleepwet, it made me so angry that I said things I don't really feel. But I wasn't angry at you. I was angry because I know how much you hate wetting when you're asleep. I'm never really angry at you inside myself, even if I yell sometimes. I'm going to try not to yell. But if I do, you'll know I don't really mean it. I love you very, very much and I know that soon you're going to be dry all night, just the way you want to be."

The bottom line is that there's no place for disciplining a child in any way in connection with sleepwetting, both because sleepwetting is unintentional and because disciplining a child for sleepwetting is likely to cause the problem to continue.

But this doesn't mean there's no place for discipline in your child's life. In fact, now is a good time for you to make sure that your overall approach to your child's behavior is what you want it to be — because if it isn't, that too can prolong sleepwetting.

The most effective disciplinary approach is to establish only rules that are reasonable and necessary, and enforce them calmly and consistently.

Establishing rules is vital so that children know exactly what is expected of them. Rules ought to be reasonable, because children only respect limits that they can make sense out of. Only necessary rules should be established, because children who are hemmed in by too many restrictions tend to become rebellious. Enforcing these rules is a must because children need to learn that at home, as in the world they'll be entering, there are limits which, if crossed, result in unpleasant consequences. Calm is crucial, because otherwise children feel they're being disciplined because a parent happens to be in a bad mood, rather than because they've broken a rule. And without consistency, children become confused about precisely where the limits are.

For instance, it's a good idea to establish a rule that a child who's had a sleepwetting incident not be allowed into the parents' bed afterwards. This rule will seem reasonable to a child if it's explained that everybody has a right to a good night's sleep in his own bed. It's a necessary rule, because parents whose privacy is disturbed by sleepwetting are going to have a hard time not expressing negative feelings about it. It can be enforced by calmly telling a child to return to his bedroom, change the wet underpad or draw-sheet, and go back to sleep. And consistency is important, because if parents give in some of the time, the child's persistence is being rewarded, and the behavior will continue.

By contrast, while a child is following the Dry All Night method, it's not a good idea to establish or enforce a rule against nail-biting, for example, or thumb-sucking. While such a rule would certainly be reasonable, for the time being it isn't necessary. In order to keep stress to a minimum, it's best to lighten up on discipline wherever resolving a problem can wait until the child becomes dry. Studies have found that children's general behavior often improves when sleepwetting is successfully treated.

In a survey of single parents, three-quarters reported that they'd become more strict after separating. They explained that because they were rushed and tired as a result of working longer hours or two jobs, and because they wanted to ward off the feeling that they were alone in a demanding world, they felt a need for more organization and control at home. "I used to be permissive with my children," one mother said, "but I no longer have the energy or time to discuss the same issue fifty-five times. So I make more rules and stick to them." If you're a single parent, this book is going to make your life easier and enable you to adopt a more relaxed attitude toward your child. So you'll probably feel less need for strictness and greater freedom to establish rules only when they're really necessary.

It's important to try to deal with other sources of stress, if they're present. For instance, if your child and a teacher aren't getting along, speak to both, and if there are valid complaints, try to deal with them. As we've seen, stress interferes with learning of every kind. Teachers know this. If you express concern that stress is getting in the way of your child's learning on all fronts, you can gain teachers' cooperation.

Your child may be having problems with peers. A child may seem gloomy, and when the parent probes, after a series of "I-don't-know" answers, the child may reluctantly admit, "I always get chosen up last to play ball." Tensions like this shouldn't be allowed to persist and interfere with attaining dryness. The child can be given sports lessons so he won't be chosen up last. And in the meantime, the parent can say, "That's okay. There are lots of things you're good at doing that other kids aren't so great at."

One common factor that can interfere with attempts to minimize stress is pressure from relatives. For example, a woman called me recently in a panic. Her mother had come to visit, and when she discovered that both her nine-year-old granddaughter and seven-year-old grandson were sleepwetters, blew up at her, insisting that she "do something" immediately. The woman, already distressed about her children's wetting, now felt she was being crowded — which made it even more difficult for her to "do something."

I asked the woman whether she used to sleepwet as a child. She said she didn't. I told her that very often, adults don't remember whether they were sleepwetting children, and I suggested that she ask her mother, just to make sure. It turned out that the woman had wet almost every night until she was seven and then gradually stopped. Once the woman's mother realized that her granddaughter's sleepwetting was something that ran in the family, rather than the result of poor parenting, the pressure stopped.

Another mother told me that her older sister was pushing her to "lower the boom" on her child — but the mother felt as if the boom was being lowered on her. If you're under this kind of pressure, I suggest that you ask friends or relatives who are worried about your child to read this book. It will assure them that you appreciate their concern, while letting them know that boom-lowering won't help. They'll realize that there's no need for them to worry, because you're doing everything that needs to be done.

No one can totally avoid stress, because it's often the result of situations beyond our control. But the stressful impact of such events can be lowered.

If a change takes place in your child's life that can cause stress — for example, the arrival of a new baby or a move to a new house — you can keep its impact to a minimum by being especially supportive.

Like many parents today, you yourself may be under a lot of stress. If you are, you'll find it relaxing to know that you're doing what needs to be done to help your child stop sleepwetting. And your child's progress in becoming dry will give you some space in which you'll be able to cope with other tensions. In the meantime, since parental stress can be a factor in causing sleepwetting, because it tends to spill over onto children, it's important to get enough sleep and exercise, and to deal with stress through techniques such as progressive relaxation, meditation, or yoga — or a walk in the park, or getting up and watching the sun rise.

The Dry All Night method's focus on encouraging the child to take responsibility for doing what's needed to stop sleepwetting is itself designed to minimize stress on both parent and child. The child is given responsibility not only in order to motivate him to achieve but to lessen any negative feelings parents may have by taking the problem off their hands. Interaction between children and parents about a subject with which neither of them is comfortable is kept to an absolute minimum. If two parents are available to handle the minimal interaction that is necessary, and one of them has strong negative feelings about sleepwetting that are difficult to deal with, it's a good idea for the other parent to take over.

Step 4: Deal with Any Contributing Factors

Give me health and a day and I will make the pomp
of emperors ridiculous.

— Emerson

As DR. DAVID SHAFFER of the College of Physicians and Surgeons of Columbia University has said, "The cause of bedwetting cannot usually be identified in an individual child." In rare instances — for example, when a child who sleepwets is also abnormally thirsty or hungry or loses weight — sleepwetting can be a sign of a medical problem. But sleepwetting is almost always just nature's way of saying that some children's bodies take a little longer to mature than others'.

A study at Tel Aviv University has found that the "bone age" of children who've never been dry, as determined from X rays, is an average of eighteen

31

months lower than their actual age. The researchers conclude that the body's night urinary control mechanism may also be "younger."

There are, however, a few conditions that can contribute to sleepwetting. So it's a good idea for your child to have a medical checkup to rule them out.

For example, if a sleepwetting child snores, the breathing difficulty may be playing a role in her sleepwetting. It's thought that the reduction in oxygen in the bloodstream caused by obstructed breathing can trigger sleepwetting incidents. Of 35 snoring children who sleepwet whose obstruction was surgically removed at Dartmouth-Hitchcock Medical Center in Hanover, New Hampshire, 26 either stopped wetting or improved.

Constipation may contribute to sleepwetting. Of 200 sleepwetting children who were examined at Minneapolis Children's Medical Center, 30 percent were constipated. A recent study found that out of 25 children referred by their doctors for further evaluation of their wetting at Montreal's Sainte-Justine Hospital, 22 were constipated. Another study has shown that 54 percent of chronically constipated children wet.

When a child has chronic constipation, researchers believe, the rectum is never completely empty. Because the rectum always contains some stool, it becomes enlarged. The enlarged rectum presses on the child's bladder. This pressure reduces the bladder's capacity and may cause it to contract. As a result, the child may wet while asleep, during the day, or both. Correcting constipation with a doctor's help can stop the wetting.

Children can be constipated without parents being aware of it. Stool that's being retained in the rectum often can't be felt by a doctor during a physical examination, and an X ray may be necessary. Both at Minneapolis Children's Medical Center and at the University of Montreal's Pediatric Research Center, 50 percent of parents of chronically constipated children had not known that their children had the problem. So if there's anything unusual about your child's bowel habits, have a talk with your doctor. Signs of chronic constipation include

- Difficulty in moving the bowels.
- Passing small, firm, dry stools.
- A child's feeling that after a bowel movement "there's something still inside."
- An interval of more than 48 hours (2 days) between bowel movements. (Though if a child has small, firm, dry stools, or feels that "not everything came out," the child is constipated no matter how often she has movements — even several times a day.)
- Passing large stools at long intervals.

- "Soiling" — that is, uncontrollable bowel movements or leakage. (Soiling, though sometimes giving the impression of being a form of diarrhea, can actually be caused by extreme constipation, as feces overflow around the hard mass that constantly remains in the rectum.)
- A series of urinary infections.

Some drugs, such as imipramine (trade name: Tofranil) and oxybutinin (trade name: Ditropan), which have been prescribed for sleepwetting (as discussed in Step 6) can have a constipating effect. If your child is chronically constipated, your doctor is unlikely to prescribe such drugs.

If the area around your child's anus itches, tell your doctor. The itching may be caused by an intestinal parasite called *Enterobius* that sometimes causes sleepwetting, particularly in girls. However, the parasite is so common that the fact that it's found in a child who sleepwets doesn't necessarily mean it is connected with the sleepwetting. Getting rid of *Enterobius* with medication takes a month, and it usually returns. So even children who've been found to have *Enterobius* should continue to use the Dry All Night method until they stop wetting.

A visit to a doctor specializing in urology is a must if your child has a urinary stream whose pressure seems too low to you, or looks too small in diameter, or comes out at an angle rather than straight; dribbles or wets during the day; or has had one or more urinary infections. (Symptoms of infection include pain or a burning sensation when urinating; an urgent need to urinate; frequent urination; pain in the lower back, lower abdomen, or pubic area; episodes of fever, weakness, tiredness, loss of appetite, nausea, or vomiting; urine that may be cloudy or dark, contain blood, or have an unusual smell.)

While urologists occasionally find a problem in the urinary system of a child who sleepwets, the two are generally unrelated. It's quite unusual, in fact, for a child with such a problem to sleepwet. And when children who do have such problems are successfully treated, only 1 out of 5 of them stops sleepwetting as a result. If surgery is recommended, more than one opinion should be obtained before proceeding.

If your child has been diagnosed as having a condition affecting water metabolism (for example, renal insufficiency), or is taking a medication that reduces kidney output (for example, desmopressin — trade name: DDAVP), the amount she drinks should be according to your doctor's instructions.

It's always reassuring for you and your child to have a talk about sleep-wetting with your pediatrician, family doctor, nurse practitioner, or physician assistant. Perhaps you've already done so. If you haven't yet, I recommend that you do. And at periodic visits, it's good to discuss your child's sleepwetting and what you've done about it. When a child finds out that her physical exam and urinalysis are just fine, stress may be reduced, speeding up the process of becoming dry all night.

Parents benefit from medical reassurance too. Any concern or anxiety that parents may feel about sleepwetting is likely to be subtly communicated to the child, causing stress that can prolong the problem. So don't sit around worrying about it — check it out!

Step 5: Communicate Supportively with Your Child

The music that can deepest reach,
And cure all ill, is cordial speech.

— Emerson

IMAGINE THAT YOU WOKE UP and found that you'd urinated while you were sleeping. You'd need all the support you could get!

Sleepwetting can make children feel pretty bad about themselves. That bad feeling can cause more sleepwetting. And more sleepwetting makes them feel still worse.

But you have the ability to break this vicious circle by supportive words and actions:

- Cheerfulness
- Expressions of affection
- Reassurance
- Encouragement
- Motivating
- Praise
- Agreement
- Attention
- Respect
- Providing opportunities for achievement

It may sound strange at first, but I believe that before long, you're going to consider yourself fortunate to have been the parent of a sleepwetting child. The most important contribution you can make to the Dry All Night method is to be as supportive to your child as possible. And being supportive to a child is the essence of being a parent — it's what we're here for. So your

34

child's sleepwetting has a silver lining: the potential to stimulate you to develop your parenting expertise to the maximum, to become the nurturing caregiver you've always known you can be.

CHEERFULNESS

Cheerfulness is necessary for supportive communication. It's hard to be supportive to someone else if you yourself are down in the dumps. But good cheer can't be faked. If you're in a bad mood, trying to sound like you're on top of the world will put you in a worse one. I hope you always feel like you just won the lottery. But even if you don't, putting this book in your child's hands, seeing her enthusiasm grow, and watching her progress is going to make you feel good and increase your ability to be cheerful when communicating with your child. It will mean a lot to her to hear you say things like, "It makes me so happy to know that you're reading your *Dry All Night* book and doing everything it says, because now I know that you're going to be dry all night very, very soon."

EXPRESSIONS OF AFFECTION

Expressions of affection are vital to helping your child become dry all night. A landmark study by a team of psychologists from Harvard, Stanford, and Cornell found that "affectional warmth" from parents was a key factor in preventing sleepwetting. Children who sleepwet need a lot of love. Of course you already show your love for your child in countless ways. But while using the Dry All Night method, it's important for you to express it in ways that children especially appreciate. A pinch on the cheek . . . a pat on the head . . . a hand around the shoulder . . . a goodnight kiss — all these show that you accept and value your child as she is, sleepwetting or no sleepwetting.

Have you hugged your sleepwetting child today?

REASSURANCE

Reassurance about anything that may be troubling your child is important. If your child ever seems upset about having had a sleepwetting episode, the first priority is to reassure her that it wasn't her fault. You can say, "It's okay. You didn't sleepwet on purpose. You didn't even know you were doing it, did you? You were fast asleep! We should never feel bad about something that happens when we're not even awake!"

In addition, tell her that lots of kids sleepwet, that it's not really a serious problem, that she's a good child who does lots of things really well — and, above all, that by following the Dry All Night method, she's doing everything she needs to do about her sleepwetting.

Children have a rather hazy idea of the future. The present absorbs them almost totally. Children who sleepwet often don't realize that just because they have this problem now doesn't mean they're always going to have it. So it's important to reassure them that their sleepwetting is only temporary by saying, "Soon you're going to stop wetting when you're asleep. Soon you're going to be dry all night."

One concept about the future that children can relate to is that of growing up. Older children and adults around them are living evidence that they won't always be small. For this reason, a powerful way for you to reassure your child is to connect becoming dry all night with growing up.

So if your child tells you she's upset because she wet during the night, an effective way of reassuring her is to say, "Right now you still wet sometimes when you're asleep, because the bladder muscle inside you is still little. But you're getting bigger every day, so your bladder is getting bigger every day, too. As soon as your bladder gets just a little bit bigger, you're going to be dry all night."

Reflecting your child's feelings back to her is a good method of reassurance. If your child is worried about sleepwetting, you can say, "Don't worry about wetting when you're asleep — I know you want to be dry all night, and soon you're going to be." Or, "I know you hate to wet when you're sleeping. That's why you're reading your *Dry All Night* book and doing everything it says so you'll stop wetting real soon."

Studies have shown that over a third of fathers and a fifth of mothers of children who sleepwet used to wet when they were children. If you used to wet, and you're comfortable talking about it, tell your child. She'll realize that sleepwetting can't be her fault if you explain to her that it's something she inherited from you, like the color of her hair or the freckles on her nose. Emphasizing that sleepwetting was a temporary problem that you got over will reassure her that sleepwetting isn't the endless grind it can sometimes seem to a young child. And letting your child know that you've "been there and back" will forge an even stronger bond between you.

If there are other things that are causing your child worry, it's important to reassure her about them also. For example, the child who's about to move to a new neighborhood needs to be reassured that she'll make new friends there. The child who's living with one parent requires frequent reassurance that the other parent still loves her and wants to be with her. The child whose parents are going through a divorce needs to be reassured that neither parent is going to abandon her. The child who's gotten a disappointing grade in a school subject needs to be reassured that, with more effort, she can do better.

It's common for children to be fearful about death, about germs, about things they've seen on TV. Reassurance for these kinds of concerns is important for children who sleepwet, because worry causes stress, and stress can prolong sleepwetting.

ENCOURAGEMENT

Encouragement is your way of expressing faith in your child, so that she'll have faith in herself. The message that needs to be conveyed is, "You can do it!" And most children who sleepwet have had at least an occasional dry night, which proves that they can.

Encouragement is important because the Dry All Night method is meant to be an easy, pleasant, and lasting method, not necessarily an instant one. Children who are eager to stop sleepwetting will be excited as they begin the Dry All Night method. But kids tend to be impatient. It's natural for them to be a little disappointed if they don't get immediate results. For your child to keep plugging away, she'll need encouragement. If you detect discouragement, you can say, "Come on, hang in there! Becoming dry all night can take a little time. Just keep reading your book every day and doing all the things it says, and soon you'll be dry all night."

In fact, this can be an opportunity for your child to learn the virtue of perseverance: not giving up until a goal is reached. By discovering that she can solve a problem by not giving up, your child can develop a character trait that will be valuable throughout her later life. When others who didn't have the "advantage" of having sleepwet as children are giving up, she'll keep on going.

Did you ever accomplish something you really wanted to do simply by refusing to give up? Was it learning to swim? To ski? To play a musical instrument? Tell your child what it was like for you. Tell her how at first you were excited to be learning something new . . . how you felt frustrated because progress didn't seem fast enough . . . how you refused to give up . . . and how it wasn't long before you achieved your goal.

MOTIVATING

Motivating means helping your child focus on how good she'll feel when she's dry all night. Motivating is made easier by the fact that you can bring into play three of the most important needs identified by one of the foremost motivational theorists, the late psychologist Dr. Abraham Maslow: affiliation, esteem, and self-actualization.

Affiliation means the need to associate with other people. You can say,

"It's going to be fun when you're dry all night, because you'll be able to sleep over at your friends' houses."

Esteem is based on feelings of competence and worthiness. You can say, "You're going to feel really good being the boss over your bladder muscle when you're sleeping."

Self-actualization is the need to be what one is meant to be, and every child is meant to be grown-up. You can say, "You're going to feel so grown-up when you're dry all night."

PRAISE

Praise your child for effort, not results. Expressions of approval of your child shouldn't be conditional on not sleepwetting — the more you express approval of your child, the more you'll have to approve of.

A good way to identify things for which you can praise your child is to make a written "asset list" of your child's strengths — character traits, personal interests, special skills, unusual achievements. The list can include clever or amusing things your child says or does. Consulting this list often and adding to it whenever possible will help you focus not only on how much you love your child but on exactly what you love about her most.

Helping a child see where she really shines is an essential element in supportive communication: "You're so good at things like playing ball and making model airplanes, you shouldn't be worrying about something that isn't your fault like wetting when you're sleeping. You're so good at doing so many things, I know that soon you'll be dry all night." Or, "You're so kind to other people, always helping them out and saying nice things to them. But when you let yourself feel bad about sleepwetting, you aren't being nice to yourself. From now on I want you to think about what a kind, sweet, grown-up person you are and never feel bad about yourself, because soon you're going to be dry all night."

AGREEMENT

Agreement is your way of confirming to your child the value of her thoughts. When your child says something you agree with, let her know it. One of the most powerful words we can say to a child is, "Right!"

ATTENTION

Attention is good for children's behavior, good for their self-image, and even good for their health. The positive impact of attention on health, in fact, is so definite that we have a scientific name for it: "attention effect." The attention effect is so pronounced that in medical experiments a "control group," which isn't receiving the treatment being tested, is often given exactly the same attention as the "treatment group." That way, if both groups improve, researchers can see how much of the improvement was caused by the specific treatment, and how much of it was the result of the attention.

What do I mean by attention? Aren't our children getting enough of it from us already? We're always chauffeuring them around, taking them shopping, serving them food, washing off their scrapes, getting their hair cut, their teeth filled, their eyes checked. What could we do for them that we aren't already doing? And besides, where can we find the time?

Parents today are busy people. So the answer isn't to increase the quantity of the attention we give our children — it's to increase the quality.

We can do this by giving our children undivided attention. We can spend time with them away from the television screen, because attention is when two people connect, not when two people stare in the same direction. We can play games with them. Fly kites with them. Go on nature walks with them. And we can just sit down and talk with them — about what's happening in their lives and ours.

Outings with just you and your child are always a good form of attention. One trip that fits nicely into the Dry All Night method is a visit to a firehouse. Part 2 will explain to your child that her bladder is like a fire truck that gets filled up with water, and that she's going to be the boss over her bladder just as the fire chief is the boss over his fire truck. When your child visits the firehouse, she can ask a fire fighter to show her a pumper truck, the kind that's featured in Part 2, and maybe even let her get inside the cab and "drive" it. Pumper trucks have water tanks inside them, so they can begin shooting water as soon as they arrive at the scene of a fire, without waiting to be connected to a hydrant, or in case there's no water source available. The tanks are usually made of fiberglass and hold between 500 and 1,000 gallons of water. If you can make time to take your child for a special, hands-on look at a pumper truck, I urge you to do so.

Because there are so many demands on parents' time, it's important to set specific "appointments" to give a child undivided attention, and stick to them. Let's put the same value on our time with our children that we do on our time with our hairdressers and exercise trainers.

When there are two parents in a household, and one of them has been less involved with a child's sleepwetting, it's a good idea for that parent to devote special attention to the child.

RESPECT

Respect from parents lets children know that the people they respect the most in the world think they're worthwhile and important. Parents can show respect for a child by asking her opinion and taking it seriously. Do you encourage your child to participate in family conversations on "adult" matters? In my experience, when young children are asked their views on family decisions, they often have useful insights to offer.

I've known parents who've told their sleepwetting child, "You're nothing but a big baby." Showing respect for a child who sleepwets means communicating the exact opposite — that the child is an emerging adult who is in the process of leaving sleepwetting behind: "You're going to be dry all night real soon, because you've got important things to do in your life, and you don't want to be bothered by wetting when you're asleep."

When we respect people, we give them the benefit of the doubt. For example, sometimes children deny having had a sleepwetting incident, despite the fact that they've obviously had one. A parent could react by saying, "Don't you lie to me!" But is that how we talk to someone we respect? Lies are meant to mislead. A person we respect would never try to mislead us. A child who denies sleepwetting isn't trying to mislead anyone — she's having a hard time coping with the hurt of sleepwetting and is trying to avoid the pain of admitting the obvious. A parent in such a situation can show respect for a child by saying, "I know it bothers you to wet when you're asleep, and you don't remember having done it, so you don't like talking about it." This shows that the parent is neither taken in by the denial nor angry at it.

PROVIDING OPPORTUNITIES FOR ACHIEVEMENT

Providing opportunities for achievement while your child is following the Dry All Night method will create an environment in which success becomes a habit. That way, becoming dry will be experienced by your child within an overall pattern of striving for personal achievement and self-fulfillment, rather than as an isolated effort to satisfy the expectations of those around her.

You can provide your child with opportunities for achievement by encouraging her to become involved in activities at which she's already shown evidence that she'll be successful. Has your child shown artistic ability? Encourage her to pick out arts and crafts materials and to make lots of projects relating to things she's interested in. You'll be able to give them the praise that they'll merit and proudly display them around the house. Has your child demonstrated skill at a particular sport? Enroll her in a league or an advanced class, so she can experience the full degree of accomplishment that's potentially hers. The child who feels competent in other areas of her life will feel competent to become dry all night.

Best of all, personally teach your child a skill she can master. I guarantee that there's something special you know how to do, something that gives you a sense of pride. I don't care whether it's weaving or astronomy, photography or magic tricks, carpentry or cartwheels — sharing that something with your child will enable both of you to experience that sense of pride together.

It's important for children to feel not only that they do things well but that they do good things. We need to help children experience the fact that they are fine, worthy, good people. We can do this by encouraging them to do acts of kindness, thoughtfulness, selflessness, and caring. The child who collects canned goods for a charity drive, or reads to a blind child, or shares her toys with poor children, will feel that she is the sort of person who deserves to be dry all night. Children naturally have an impulse to do things like these. But they need us as facilitators, to put them in touch with opportunities not just to feel good about themselves but to feel that they themselves are good.

Some people are better at doing things than others. But everybody has the ability to do better things!

And finally, supportiveness begins at home. To be truly supportive to your child, you've got to be supportive to yourself. One of the best ways you can help your child achieve her goal of becoming dry all night is to make this a time of setting goals for yourself and achieving them. Learn . . . create . . . excel . . . form new relationships . . . act on your ideals . . . show your compassion for people outside your usual circle. Be caring toward yourself as if you were your own child, and you'll be better able to help your child move not just toward dryness but toward a fulfilling adulthood.

Step 6: Be Careful about Drugs for Sleepwetting

Every sweet has its sour . . .

— Emerson

A NUMBER OF DRUGS have been given for sleepwetting with varying effectiveness, and your doctor may wish to try one with your child. If so, there's no conflict between using a medication and following the method presented in Part 2. For example, manufacturers of imipramine offer it as a "temporary adjunctive therapy" for sleepwetting. "Adjunctive" means "something joined or added to another thing but not essentially a part of it." So it shouldn't be used alone, but only in combination with other steps.

If your doctor prescribes medication, make sure you're clear on exactly how long your child is supposed to take it. Imipramine, for instance, is usually given for a maximum of three months. All in all, says Dr. Stephen A. Koff, of the Ohio State University College of Medicine, Division of Urology, "Considering the potential and unknown risks of long-term pharmacotherapy, drugs such as imipramine probably should be reserved for failures of other therapy or when short-term dry periods are essential."

Medication can provide a child with a period during which there are fewer wetting episodes or even none. Such a "dry spell" may help by breaking the cycle of wetting → stress → wetting → stress → wetting. By showing a child that it isn't impossible for him to be dry, cutting this negative-feedback loop can set the stage for lasting improvement.

But because no drug "cures" sleepwetting, when your doctor takes your child off medication it's extremely important that your child not stop following the Dry All Night method. Your child should continue reading Part 2 and following its instructions.

Here is information on three drugs that have been prescribed for sleepwetting.

IMIPRAMINE

The standard drug guide for physicians, *Goodman and Gilman's The Pharmaceutical Basis of Therapeutics,* states regarding imipramine (trade name: Tofranil): "Enuresis [sleepwetting] in children over 6 years of age has been accepted as a possible use for imipramine, but such treatment produces only temporary effects."

Imipramine is quite toxic compared to other drugs, causing side effects in as many as 1 in 20 people. In rare instances, imipramine causes a dangerous blood condition called granulocytopenia. Children taking the drug should have a blood test every few weeks. If your child feels ill, or develops a sore throat or sore mouth, fever, chills, or weakness while on imipramine, the drug should be stopped, and you should immediately take your child to the doctor for a blood test. Imipramine shouldn't be taken by a child with a heart problem, and it's been recommended that all children have electrocardiograms before and while receiving it.

One possible side effect of imipramine is constipation. As we saw in Step 4, constipation can contribute to sleepwetting. So if your child becomes constipated, tell your doctor.

Because sleepwetting is physically harmless, parents often assume that any drug used to treat it must be harmless too. But tablet-for-tablet, imipramine is one of the more toxic drugs on the market. Children being treated for sleepwetting, as well as their brothers and sisters, have accidentally been poisoned — some of them fatally. So if your doctor prescribes imipramine, take the following precautions:

- Make sure a minimum number of tablets is dispensed at any one time.
- Double-check that the container in which the drug is kept is correctly labeled and has a child-resistant closure that works.
- Tell your child how many tablets to take at one time; explain that taking more could make him very sick.
- Explain that he should never take any medication unless you are in the room.
- Never refer to any medication as "candy."
- Keep the tablets out of children's reach, preferably under lock and key.
- Be aware of the symptoms of imipramine poisoning, which may include reddening of the skin, dry mouth, rapid heartbeat, restlessness, confusion, loss of muscular control, enlarged pupils, urine retention, fever, convulsions, paralysis, coma, rapid breathing, respiratory arrest, and cardiac arrest.
- Post poison control center telephone numbers.
- Have a one-ounce (29.5 milliliter) bottle of ipecac syrup U.S.P. you can give to induce vomiting.
- Flush remaining imipramine down the toilet when your child is taken off it.

OXYBUTININ

Oxybutinin (trade name: Ditropan) and other "anticholinergic" medications are often prescribed for children who also have daytime urinary symptoms — uncontrolled wetting, frequent urination, or a feeling that they must urinate urgently. It is far less toxic than imipramine, though it too can have side effects, and an overdose is dangerous.

Watch for constipation, a possible side effect of oxybutinin, which can contribute to sleepwetting.

Oxybutinin reduces sweating, so if your doctor prescribes it, make sure your child isn't exposed to a hot environment, which could cause potentially fatal heat stroke. Ask your doctor to familiarize you with the signs of heat stroke and first-aid measures for it.

43

DESMOPRESSIN

Desmopressin (trade name: DDAVP) was developed to reduce urinary output in people with a form of diabetes. Because it acts immediately, though temporarily, it could be useful when a dry night is important, such as an overnight school trip.

Desmopressin has few side effects. But consult your doctor about how much your child should drink during the hours that the drug is active. Since desmopressin temporarily lowers the amount of water excreted by the kidneys, drinking more than enough to satisfy thirst can result in water intoxication.

Step 7: Help Your Child Make a Dry All Night Scoreboard

The reward of a thing well done, is to have done it.

— Emerson

AS YOU'LL SEE IN PART 2, your child is being given responsibility for keeping a record of her progress by drawing pictures on a "scoreboard" with a column for each day of the week. Psychologists call this technique "self-monitoring." When a child is given complete responsibility, any achievement will belong completely to her. The sense of achievement your child will feel from watching her own progress, as charted by her on her own scoreboard, will be her main "reward" for following the Dry All Night method.

Because of the importance of your child's taking personal responsibility for doing away with sleepwetting, if she's able to make the blank scoreboard completely on her own she should be encouraged to do so. Unless more help is necessary, all you'll do is make sure she has everything she needs — paper, writing instruments, and a ruler. You can say, "I think you'll have fun making your Dry All Night scoreboard and drawing on it. Your scoreboard is going to help you become dry all night."

If your child wants to draw additional charts herself, by all means encourage her to do so. But often it will be most convenient if your child makes one "master" scoreboard in black marker, pen, or pencil to be photocopied as necessary. The size of the master should depend on the type of copier you have access to. If the copier takes large paper, the master can be made on paper that size, as big as possible. If it's capable of enlarging originals, the master can be made in any size.

Dry All Night SCOREBOARD

Week beginning: _____
Month / Day

I want to be DRY ALL NIGHT this week because: _____

	Sunday	Monday	Tuesday	Wednesday	Thursday	Friday	Saturday
I was DRY ALL NIGHT last night !							
This afternoon I drank a great big glass of powerful H_2O							
Then I sat on my bed and read my DRY ALL NIGHT book							

It's good for your child to do as much of the actual copying process as possible with her own hands. If you have access to a copier that your child can operate, encourage your child to carry the original to the place where the copier is, put the master in the machine, press the button, take the copies and original out, and carry them home. If the only place you can make copies is at a store where a clerk operates the machine, don't bring your child with you, so that she won't be embarrassed.

This is one case where neatness does not count — as long as the necessary spaces are there, the scoreboard is fine, even if the lines aren't so straight. Similarly, the Dry All Night scoreboard isn't a spelling bee — as long as your child can make sense out of what she's written, let any mistakes go by.

Even if you think your child is too young to make the blank scoreboard all by herself, encourage her to try — she may surprise you. If it turns out that she has difficulty making the scoreboard, it's time for you (in a two-parent household, preferably the parent who's previously been less involved with the child's sleepwetting) to ask her if she'd like some help. Helping her only after she expresses her desire for your assistance is the way to give her a hand without taking away from her feeling of responsibility. If she does need help, don't jump in and draw the scoreboard for her. Sit down next to her, let her begin, praise her as she goes along, and only draw or write on the paper when you have to. Even drawing only a single line or writing a single word will increase her feeling of accomplishment.

I've included a blank version of the sample scoreboard that appears in Part 2. You'll find it on page 45. If your child has difficulty making her own master scoreboard, and you can't spare the time to help her with it, she can photocopy this one.

Your child can put her Dry All Night scoreboard wherever she wants to. She'll probably want it to be in a place where friends, brothers, sisters, adult relatives, and other visitors won't see it unless she lets them — for example, the inside of her closet door, or a desk drawer. You can say, "It'll be fun to put your scoreboard where only you and I can look at it." Some children will want to show their scoreboard to others as they fill it in — your child may positively drag people to look at it. Other children will treat their scoreboard as something very personal and private. If so, help them keep it that way.

Make sure your child has a supply of washable markers with plenty of life in them, or not-too-short, sharpened crayons or colored pencils. Bringing a child a new set of markers, crayons, or colored pencils "as a present for drawing on your Dry All Night scoreboard," or taking her to a store to pick out a new set, will encourage her to begin filling in her chart.

If your child goes to stay overnight at the home of a noncustodial or shared-custody parent, make sure she takes the scoreboard she's filling in with her. She should bring plenty of drawing materials, as well as a supply of blank scoreboards.

At the beginning of the week, your child will have an opportunity to write the most important reason why she wants to be dry all night in the space provided on her scoreboard. This allows children to focus on what their main motivation for becoming dry is, to change it if they want to, and to remind themselves of it if it's still the same. Some children will write something like, "So I don't have to sleep in a wet bed anymore." Others will write, "So I can sleep over at my friend's house." Others may not feel like writing anything. If yours doesn't, don't push her.

Your child is going to draw a picture of a glass of water every time she drinks "a great big glass of H_2O," as she'll be asked to do each afternoon just before reading Part 2. After she reads Part 2, she'll draw a picture of her *Dry All Night* book. Drawing these pictures will allow her to use her creativity in recording her progress. Looking at them will give her a feeling of accomplishment by showing her that she is doing the things that will help her become dry all night. As described in Step 9, by looking at your child's scoreboard you'll be able to confirm that your child is reading Part 2 and following its instructions. (Occasionally, a child doesn't want to draw on the scoreboard. If your child doesn't want to, you can take her to a store and let her pick out and pay for stickers to put in the boxes instead of drawing in them.)

Whenever your child has a night in which she didn't wet while she was asleep, she'll draw a picture of Dan the Magic Camel, Christopher's guide in Part 2. The best time for your child to draw the picture is right after she gets up, when her enthusiasm about being dry is at its highest. It's a good idea for you not to check your child's bed as soon as she wakes up to see whether or not she was dry. If the bed is wet, you may find yourself inadvertently expressing negative feelings. It's wiser to wait until your child is out of the room — even better, out of the house — before you check.

If your child asks you to look at her scoreboard, take the opportunity to reinforce her sense of personal achievement. You can say, "I bet it makes you feel really good to look at your scoreboard and see all the things you're doing all by yourself to become dry all night."

Or: "Look at all those glasses of water and books. It's really great the way you're doing all the things you need to do to be dry all night."

Or: "Hey, there's a camel! You were dry all night! Wow! You know something? Soon you're going to be dry all night all the time!"

If your child tells you that she wet while she was sleeping, it's important to reassure and encourage her. You can give her a big hug and tell her, "That's okay. It wasn't your fault — after all, it happened when you were fast asleep! And you can be really proud of yourself for reading your *Dry All Night* book and doing what it says to do. Keep on reading your book every day and doing everything it says to do, and soon you're going to be dry all night."

If your child tells you that she didn't wet, congratulations are in order. You can give her a big hug and say, "That's great. Reading your *Dry All Night* book and doing everything it says to do really helps, doesn't it? Soon you're going to be dry all night all the time."

I'm often asked whether I'm in favor of material rewards for dry nights. My answer is that just as children shouldn't be punished for something they did while they were sleeping, they shouldn't be rewarded for something they didn't do while they were sleeping. I tell parents that giving a child a shiny new quarter for having a dry night is about as logical as giving a child a shiny new quarter for growing an inch.

Because children are used to being rewarded only for desirable actions that they perform deliberately, and punished only for undesirable actions that they perform deliberately, to reward a child for dry nights would imply that you believe that any wet nights must have been deliberate. This would cause stress, and stress can prolong sleepwetting.

Dangling a big-ticket reward in front of a child for stopping wetting completely can actually be counterproductive. I've known of cases in which parents have said that when their children stopped, they'd buy them their own video, or even take them to Disney World. The grand-prize approach didn't work. The kids weren't as eager to hit the jackpot as they were worried that they wouldn't. And not receiving the reward felt like a punishment. In my experience, buying a child who sleepwets a new bike, with no strings attached, is more likely to help her become dry all night than promising to buy her one when she becomes dry.

Even for actions the child can control, such as following the steps in Part 2, material rewards, such as toys, candy, and money, should be kept to a minimum. When a parent offers a material reward to a child for desired behavior, it can make the child feel that the parent is offering her a "bribe" because the parent doesn't trust her to do what she's supposed to. Instead of encouraging a child, this can actually discourage her. Material rewards foster a "what's-in-it-for-me" attitude that may remain after sleepwetting is long forgotten. What behavioral psychologists call "evaluative reinforcement" — words of praise — can be a far more meaningful reward to your child than a candy bar. Telling your child, "It's really great the way you've been reading your *Dry All Night* book and doing all the things it says to do," is not a less effective means of reinforcement than giving her a Twinkie.

Children love surprises, and a wonderful way to reward a child is to take her off guard — especially with an offer of quality time: "You know, you've been so grown-up about reading your *Dry All Night* book and doing all the things it says to do — it makes me feel so good that I want to just be with you. How about picking a game and we'll play it together."

Some children do need an extra push, and if yours is one of them, you can offer a special treat. You can say, "You know what I think? I think that from now on, you're going to read your *Dry All Night* book every day and do everything it says, so you'll be dry all night, like you want to be. And then you know what I'm going to do? I'm going to take you to the zoo!"

But your child's basic reward for following the steps in Part 2 should be the sense of responsibility she'll feel when she sees by the glasses of water and books she's drawn that she's been doing what she needs to do to be dry all night — and the sense of achievement she'll feel as she sees a caravan of magic camels begin to cross her Dry All Night scoreboard.

Once your child has gone at least three weeks without wetting while asleep — 21 camels in a row — she can start drinking as much as she feels like after supper, rather than only drinking if she feels "pretty thirsty" (as she's asked to do in Part 2). If she has no further wet nights, after at least three more weeks — 21 more dry nights, for a total of at least six dry weeks — she can stop reading Part 2 and following its steps.

After beginning to drink after supper without being "pretty thirsty," your child may start to have some accidents. This is completely normal, and there's no need for her to cut back on drinking after supper. She should simply continue reading Part 2 and following its steps until she has had at least another 21 consecutive dry nights. After these additional three weeks of being dry all night, she can "graduate" from the Dry All Night method.

It's unlikely that after "graduating," your child will begin to have a series of "accidents," but it's possible. It could happen months later, or even years later. If so, it's nothing to be alarmed about. Reassure your child, giving her a big hug and telling her, "Don't worry. Your bladder muscle has just forgotten a little bit about what it's supposed to do. You're going to read your *Dry All Night* book again and do everything it says, to remind your bladder muscle exactly what to do. Soon you're going to be dry all night all the time." Your child should begin reading Part 2 again, following its steps until she's been dry for three weeks while drinking after supper only when "pretty thirsty," and for another three weeks while drinking as much as she feels like.

Step 8: Know Why Drinking Plenty of Water Will Help

Everything in Nature contains all the powers of Nature.

— Emerson

PARENTS OFTEN TRY TO DEAL with sleepwetting by limiting how much their children drink. But research has shown that restricting fluids doesn't help, and can actually delay improvement.

In fact, we now know that drinking freely during the day actually increases children's ability to hold urine while they're sleeping. So Part 2 of this book is going to encourage your child to drink "plenty of powerful H_2O" — good old nonfattening, non–tooth-decaying water — during the daytime, while drinking only when "pretty thirsty" after supper.

Research studies at such centers as Baltimore's Johns Hopkins University School of Medicine, Harvard Medical School, the University of Saskatchewan, and Northwestern University Medical School, have found that "functional bladder capacity" — the term used by urologists for the amount of urine a child can hold in his bladder before he feels that he has to urinate — is usually lower in children who sleepwet than in children the same age who don't wet.

This doesn't mean that your child's bladder is smaller than it should be — just that, right now, it isn't holding as much as it should.

In a study at the Medical College of Wisconsin in Milwaukee, a team of urologists found that whenever children who sleepwet urinated, whether they were asleep or awake, the amount that came out — their functional bladder capacity — was lower than that of children who didn't sleepwet. Did this mean that the actual physical capacity of their bladders was lower?

To find out, the researchers used a technique known as "cystometry." Under general anesthesia, they filled the children's bladders with water through a tube. The actual physical capacity of the bladders of children who wet turned out to be exactly the same as that of children who didn't wet. And the actual physical bladder capacity of the children who sleepwet was two to three times as much as their functional capacity. So the problem was that their bladders were simply not holding as much as they were physically capable of holding.

What can be done to increase a child's functional bladder capacity?

In a landmark experiment, Dr. T.-B. Hagglund, of Children's Castle, the famed pediatric hospital in Helsinki, Finland, divided a number of sleepwetting children with ages ranging up to thirteen into two groups. One group was repeatedly instructed not to drink anything at all in the evening. The other was urged to drink more than normally during the day. By the end of the experimental period, the fluid-restriction group's average functional bladder capacity had gone down by 9 percent. None of the children had stopped wetting, while 17 percent were wetting less often.

The children in the second group were offered tasty drinks during the day and urged to drink more than they normally would. Other than that, they received no special handling. By the end of the experiment, the group's average functional bladder capacity had gone up by 20 percent, 33 percent of the children had stopped sleepwetting completely, and 39 percent were wetting less often.

The "increase of bladder capacity that can be observed after a period of [greater-than-normal] drinking with wetting ignored," Dr. Hagglund commented, "is probably due to the decrease of the tonus and irritability of the bladder musculature.

"The very satisfactory results of [greater-than-normal] drinking and the negative effect of fluid restriction on the enuretic symptom and bladder-emptying mechanism," said Dr. Hagglund, "are probably due to both the physiological effect of the fluid on the bladder and perhaps more to the psychological significance such a form of treatment has. When an enuretic child is allowed to drink plenty of fluid and to play with it, and when the feeling of shame about the wetting is eliminated, then the earlier stress and psychic tension attached to the symptom will diminish, and at the same time the tension and irritability of the bladder will lessen."

Or, as Dr. Barton D. Schmitt of the pediatrics department at the University of Colorado Health Sciences Center, Denver, says, "More fluid intake means more urine production. More urine leads to larger bladders [in terms of functional capacity]."

The Dry All Night method emphasizes drinking water because many other liquids children commonly drink have been implicated in causing sleepwetting. For example, cocoa and chocolate contain a chemical called theobromine that increases the flow of urine from the kidneys. Cola drinks and tea contain caffeine, which has the same effect.

Plus, you don't have to lug water home, it doesn't take up space in the fridge, you don't have to open it, mix it, thaw it, or squeeze it, and the price is right. And since it's important that your child drink in the daytime, it has the advantage that, unlike most other beverages, it comes out of a pipe at school.

In addition to encouraging your child to drink lots of water during the day, Part 2 will tell him to drink "a great big glass" before reading its picture story each afternoon. Your child will be told that after he finishes reading, he should go to the bathroom and urinate. This step is included because of the importance of what Drs. Sumner H. Marshall, Hermine H. Marshall, and Richards P. Lyon, of the University of California School of Medicine and Division of Educational Psychology, have called "sensation awareness." These researchers have emphasized that a child who sleepwets "needs to become aware of a full bladder and of the necessity to void when these sensations are experienced. If he is aware of his own bodily sensations, he will often realize that he can control them — that he can be master of his own body." Dr. James M. Stedman, of the University of Texas Medical School at San Antonio, has called this principle "bladder awareness."

It's clear that during the daytime, your child (and this includes children who wet during the day also) should be drinking plentifully. But what about the hours between supper and bedtime?

Even adults who've had an unusually large amount to drink shortly before bedtime may sometimes find themselves being awakened in the middle of the night by the urge to go to the bathroom. For children, drinking a lot before going to sleep is asking for trouble. So after your child eats supper, liquids should be discouraged.

Discouraged — but not prohibited. We've seen that stopping fluids in the evening is actually counterproductive, decreasing the functional bladder capacity that we want to increase. Restricting fluids can also make a child feel that you don't believe he'll be able to control his bladder while he's sleeping — that the only way he can stop fluid from coming out is to stop it from coming in. But above all, children should always be able to quench their thirst, 24 hours a day.

Your child will be asked in Part 2 not to drink after supper unless "pretty thirsty." Trust your child. If you see him drinking after supper, assume that he really needs to, and don't say anything about it. Of course it's possible that he could be drinking more than he absolutely must. But it's not worth having an argument over. Unnecessary tension is much worse for a child who sleepwets than unnecessary liquids!

If your child is used to having a bedtime glass of milk, now is a good time to phase it out. You can explain that grownups don't have anything to drink right before they go to bed either, because they want to be dry all night, just the way he does.

Parents often tell me that their sleepwetting child takes a bottle to bed. I'm a big believer in security blankets, favorite pillows, indispensable dolls, necessary teddy bears, and — for children who don't wet — nighttime bottles. But children who sleepwet should switch to hanging onto something that isn't filled with liquid. You can gently tell a child who's been sleeping with a bottle, "I know it makes you feel good to have a bottle at night. But not having a bottle at night will help you become dry all night, which will make you feel even better. What would you like to take to bed with you from now on instead of a bottle?"

My recommendation, in a nutshell: "A lot more to drink during the daytime, a little less to drink after supper — and a visit to the john before getting into bed."

Step 9: Minimize Verbal Reminders about Following Part 2

Self-reliance, the height and perfection of man . . .

— Emerson

THE STUDY CONDUCTED BY Drs. Marshall, Marshall, and Lyon of the University of California found that when a child takes responsibility for becoming dry at night, the results are more successful than when parents try to do things "for" a child.

This makes sense in the light of one of the fundamental principles of child psychology: the most important factor motivating children is the desire for "mastery," also known as "competence," "self-efficacy," and "autonomous achievement." Put simply, we know that children want to be able to do things — not to have things done to them.

And, as indicated by that word "autonomous," they don't just want to do things — they want to be the ones to do them! If your child went through a stage, as a toddler, in which she wanted to do things all by herself, you know exactly what I'm talking about. Each of my children not only insisted on doing things "by self" — if I dared to try to help them in the slightest way during this amusing but exasperating phase, they wouldn't be satisfied until they were able to do the task all over again, this time totally on their own.

The desire for mastery in older children isn't expressed by demands for "do-overs." And it's joined by such new motivations as the desire for acceptance by peers. But it's just as strong. Your child's natural desire for mastery is her most powerful motivation to do away with sleepwetting. You want to harness that power. So it's vital not to do anything that would lessen your child's sense that becoming dry all night is her own responsibility — so that she'll know that when she stops wetting, it will be her own accomplishment. The way for you to encourage this all-important feeling of taking complete personal responsibility is to keep verbal reminders to a minimum.

In plain English: Don't nag!

Direct oral reminders by parents can backfire. It's been found that children actually tend to stop following programs designed to deal with their problems if parents repeatedly tell them to follow the programs. Children are not going to get behind the wheel and head for a destination — even a destination they really want to get to — if parents insist on being backseat drivers.

One of the primary purposes of this book, therefore, is to provide a program that is self-reminding. The book, not the parent, is the reminder.

Part 2 will make it clear to your child that the way to become dry all night is to read it every day and do everything it says to do. Rather than asking her whether she's doing so, just check your child's Dry All Night scoreboard every few days. By seeing whether your child is drawing books and glasses of water on her scoreboard regularly, you'll know if she's following the method.

Another way of keeping tabs on your child's taking responsibility is to keep an eye on the night-lights in your child's bedroom and in the bathroom where she'll be urinating. Part 2 will tell your child to turn on a "little light" in the bathroom after she urinates just before getting into bed, and another in her bedroom just before she gets into bed. These night-lights — as well as a night-light on the way to the bathroom, if the path isn't otherwise lit — are important in themselves, because many children are afraid of the dark, and it's helpful to remove any possible causes of reluctance to get out of bed and go to the bathroom.

They can also be useful as a means of encouraging your child to take responsibility. You can take your child to a store where she can pick out inexpensive night-lights — if she wishes, in the shape of her favorite cartoon characters — take them to the cashier, pay for them, and receive the change. She can decide exactly which outlets they should be plugged into. And turning them on at night and off in the morning will be her "job."

By quietly checking to see whether both lights are on after she has gotten into bed, you'll know whether she's followed this step. If one or more lights are not on, and she's still awake, you can say, "You know what? I think you forgot to put your little light(s) on, the way it says to do in your *Dry All Night* book. I bet you want to put your little light(s) on right now, to help you be dry all night." If the night-light is off in the bathroom, it may mean that she didn't urinate before getting into bed. You can say, "Sometimes I forget to urinate into the toilet right before I get into bed. Maybe you forgot tonight. When you turn on your little light in the bathroom, it's a good time for you to remember to put your urine in the toilet, where you want it to go. Urinating into the toilet before you get in bed is going to help you be dry all night."

If there are two parents in the household, the best approach is for the parent who has previously had less to do with the child's sleepwetting to monitor her progress — and, if absolutely necessary, to remind her.

Most children will quickly and smoothly get into the habit of reading and following Part 2. But if by some chance you see that your child isn't getting into it, don't speak to her about it unless you have to. Instead, use the book as the reminder:

- Before your child comes home from school (which may mean before you leave for work), put *Dry All Night* on the table or desk where she does her homework.
- If your child arrives home before you do, put *Dry All Night* where you leave messages or snacks for her.
- After your child is asleep, gently check to see if she has put *Dry All Night* under her pillow, as she is asked to do in Part 2. If she hasn't, get the book and quietly put it there. If while you're checking you see that she has awakened, you can say, "I'm going to put your *Dry All Night* book under your pillow so you'll remember to be dry all night." (It's a good idea for you to have an additional copy of this book on your own bookshelf so that if you don't find your child's copy under her pillow, you won't have to search for it. In the morning, you can locate your child's copy and return your own copy to your shelf.)
- If your child regularly spends the night at the home of a noncustodial parent, shared-custody parent, or other relative, don't remind her to take *Dry All Night* with her. Put the book in her bag without saying anything about it. Or better, since there's always the possibility that she may forget to bring the book home with her, arrange for there to be another copy of *Dry All Night* at the relative's house, and explain to the relative, in a private conversation, how to use it as a reminder if necessary.

In most cases, using the book itself as a reminder will do the trick. If it doesn't, write a note to your child and leave it for her in a sealed envelope with her name and address on the outside. The note can say something like

> Dear ———,
> Because you're getting so grown-up, here's a grown-up letter to help you remember to read your *Dry All Night* book every afternoon and to do everything it says so that you'll be dry all night real soon.
>
> Love,
Mommy or Daddy

If no drawings appear on her scoreboard, you can write to her a few times. Sometimes even adults need to receive several written reminders before they take action!

If you still don't see any action on your child's scoreboard, don't get angry. Don't yell. Don't groan. Don't tsk. Don't threaten. Don't complain. Don't beg. Sit down with her in a quiet place when both you and she are rested and in a good mood, and have a heart-to-heart.

Begin the conversation with a hug and a kiss. If your lap can stand the wear and tear, sit her on it. If not, put your arm around her shoulder. Ask her to tell you how she feels about reading her *Dry All Night* book and doing the things it says to do. Then tell her, very softly, something like this:

"Dry All Night is your book, not mine, and I don't want to be reminding you all the time to read it and to do all the things it says. Just the way I wouldn't like you to have to remind me all the time to do something. After all, you're the one who doesn't like wetting when you're asleep. And you're the one who wants to do something about it.

"But I love you so much that I want to make sure that just because you're such a busy kid with so many things to do, you don't forget to read Part 2 every afternoon and to do everything it says, because I know how much you want to be dry all night."

While you're going to speak to your child about Part 2 only as a last resort, if she brings the subject up by all means feel free to talk with her about it. There's no problem in talking about Part 2 with your child, as long as you're not the one who starts the conversation. Because if she's the one who comes to you about it, that will mean she's taking responsibility for following the Dry All Night method.

A few children exhibit a general behavior pattern we call "oppositional." Whatever we want them to do, they seem to want to do the opposite. Their favorite word is "no." They're contrary. They argue. They're stubborn. When they don't get their way, they dig their heels in and may even throw a tantrum. If your child is oppositional, it isn't because she's "bad." Her inborn desire for mastery and autonomy has simply led her into conflict with people around her. She has yet to learn that getting into unnecessary conflict with other people isn't an effective way of expressing mastery over herself.

If your child is oppositional, the last thing you want to do is get into a power struggle with her. Such a battle of wills can only escalate until it's won by the more powerful individual: you. But the child will still be left with the same need for mastery — which just means you'll have to fight a rematch at a time and place of her choosing.

Better to use "reverse psychology." If a child says, "I don't want to read that book. I don't want to read any books," don't fall into the trap of saying,

"You'll read that book or else." The best thing for you to say is, "That's fine with me. I've changed my mind. I've decided I don't want you to read it after all. It's for grown-up kids, and I thought it was for you, because sometimes you act like you're really grown up. But if you don't want to read it every day, it means you aren't grown-up enough yet. I know you'll be grown-up enough very soon, but right now I can see that you aren't, so you shouldn't read the book and you shouldn't do all the grown-up things it says to do." At that point, the way for the oppositional child to show who's in charge will be — to insist on reading the book and doing every last thing it says!

Step 10: Give This Book to Your Child as a Present

The only gift is a portion of thyself.

— Emerson

THIS IS THE LAST STEP in Part 1. After you've finished Part 1, read Part 2 if you haven't already read it, so you'll know exactly what your child will be doing. Then, if you bought your copy of *Dry All Night,* or received it as a gift, wrap it in decorative paper and make a special point of giving it to your child as a present. Tying it up with a ribbon or sticking on a ready-made bow will make it even more fun for your child to receive. Most important is a personal card or note from you, saying something like, "Here's a special present I got just for you. This book is going to help you to be dry all night."

When your child opens up his present, tell him, "You know what this is? It's a special book called *Dry All Night* that's going to help you stop wetting when you're asleep. You can read it again and again and again. I think you're going to have lots of fun reading it every afternoon.

"Now that you're getting so grown-up, you can do special things that will help you stop wetting when you're asleep. When you read your new *Dry All Night* book, you're going to find out all the things you can do. You're going to be able to do the things all by yourself. I think you're going to have lots of fun doing all the things the book shows you how to do. Doing all the things in your book will help you be dry all night, real soon."

If you borrowed your copy, of course you won't gift-wrap it. But do tell your child that you got it especially for him, that you think he'll have fun doing all the things it says to do, and that doing all the things it says to do will help him be dry all night.

The basic idea of the Dry All Night method is to put in children's hands a step-by-step guide to becoming dry that they'll find interesting and entertaining — and will therefore require as little effort by parents as possible. Exactly how little effort will depend on a number of factors — the child's age, level of maturity, motor skills, and so forth. But one thing is clear: the more your child relates to this book, the more readily he'll take responsibility for becoming dry. Letting your child know that *Dry All Night* belongs to him will encourage him to read Part 2 and follow its steps.

If your child reads with difficulty or is dyslexic, suggest to him that when he reads Part 2, he may find it easier and more understandable if he reads it out loud. If this doesn't help enough, you can make a cassette tape of the text of Part 2, which your child can play while looking at the pictures.

The best voice to use on such a tape is the child's own. (If your child doesn't read aloud well enough, and there are two parents in your household, the voice of the parent who's less involved with his sleepwetting should be on the tape. A tape with the voice of a grandparent, or an aunt or uncle the child is close to, is also good. It's best not to use the voice of a brother or sister, since children can be sensitive about other children's awareness of their wetting.)

I wouldn't recommend that Part 2 be read to your child "live," because it's so important that children take responsibility for helping themselves to stop wetting, with a minimum of assistance from others. But if your child asks you to read Part 2 to him, it's fine for you to do it, because he's the one who's taking the initiative.

Once they know the story, many children will just skim the text of Part 2, and concentrate on the pictures.

A CONCLUDING ADDRESS

Receiving letters from parents who've used *Toilet Learning* has given me tremendous satisfaction. Now I look forward with great anticipation to hearing from you about your experiences in helping your child become dry all night. (If you'll enclose a filled-in Dry All Night scoreboard that you've asked your child for so you can send it to me, I'll put it up on a special wall in my house.)

And I'm especially hopeful that I'll be getting other letters, too. I've received many photos of children who've used *Toilet Learning*. Usually they're snapped while the child is sitting on the toilet, reading it. One of the cutest potty pictures, showing two-year-old Chelsea Clair of Napa, California, even won a blue ribbon at the local county fair! But *Toilet Learning* was for toddlers. Which means that I've never received a letter from a child about it. So I can't wait to hear from children who'd like to receive a note from a real live author, thanking them for reading her book — and for becoming dry all night.

My address is

Alison Mack
DRY ALL NIGHT
350 West 57 St.
New York, NY 10019

Part 2

For Children

Soon I'll Be Dry All Night!

Erin and Brandi were best friends.

They went to school together. They went to the mall together. They went everywhere together.

They rode bikes together. They played together. They did everything together.

One day Brandi said, "I'd like you to stay overnight at my house, Erin. We can eat together. We can read books together. We can watch TV together. And best of all, we can sleep in the same room!"

"I'd love to!" said Erin.

"Great, " said Brandi. "Let's do it tonight."

Erin felt good. She always wanted to sleep over at Brandi's house. She was very happy.

But then she remembered . . .

"I don't think I can do it tonight," Erin said.

"That's okay," said Brandi. "How about tomorrow night?"

"I don't think my mom will let me," said Erin.

"Sure she will," Brandi said. "Come on — we'll have fun!"

"I don't know. Maybe some other time." Erin felt like she was going to cry. "I think I'd better go home now," Erin said.

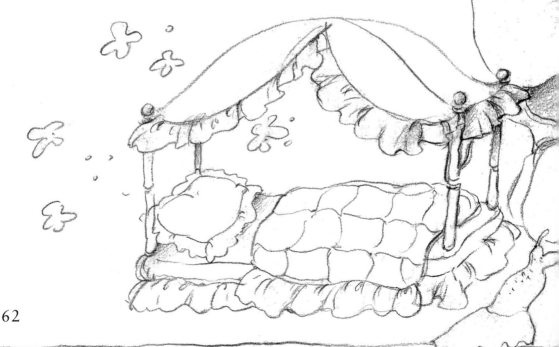

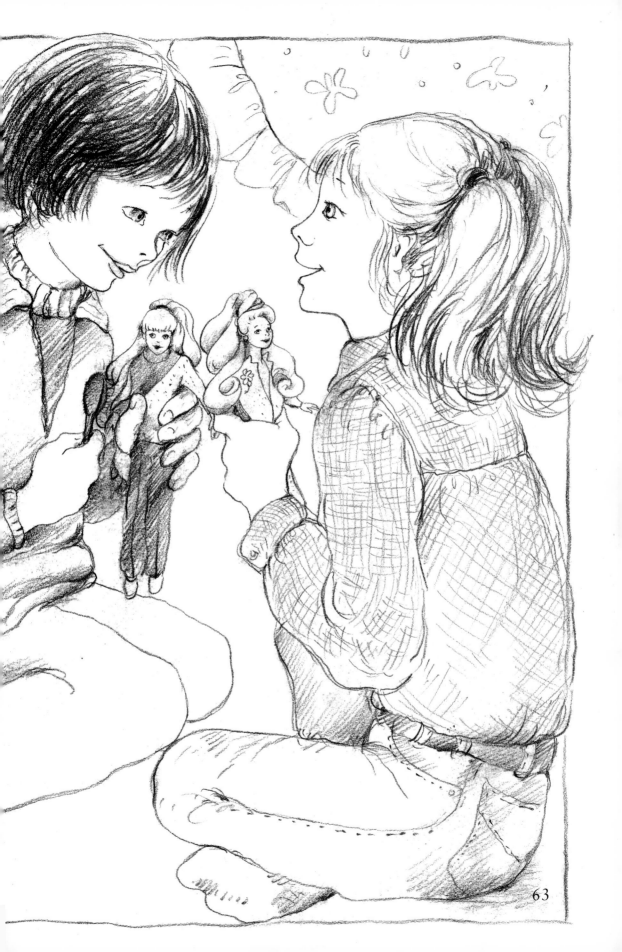

63

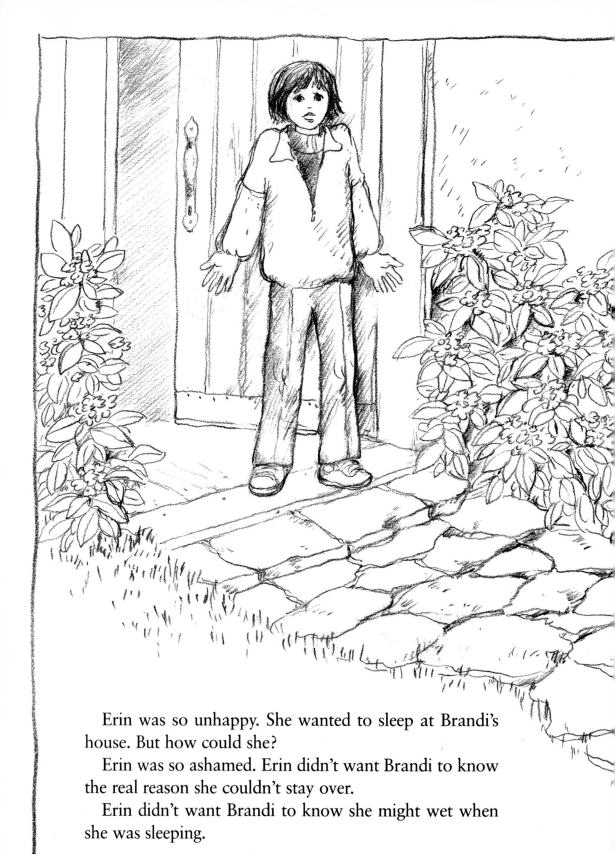

Erin was so unhappy. She wanted to sleep at Brandi's house. But how could she?

Erin was so ashamed. Erin didn't want Brandi to know the real reason she couldn't stay over.

Erin didn't want Brandi to know she might wet when she was sleeping.

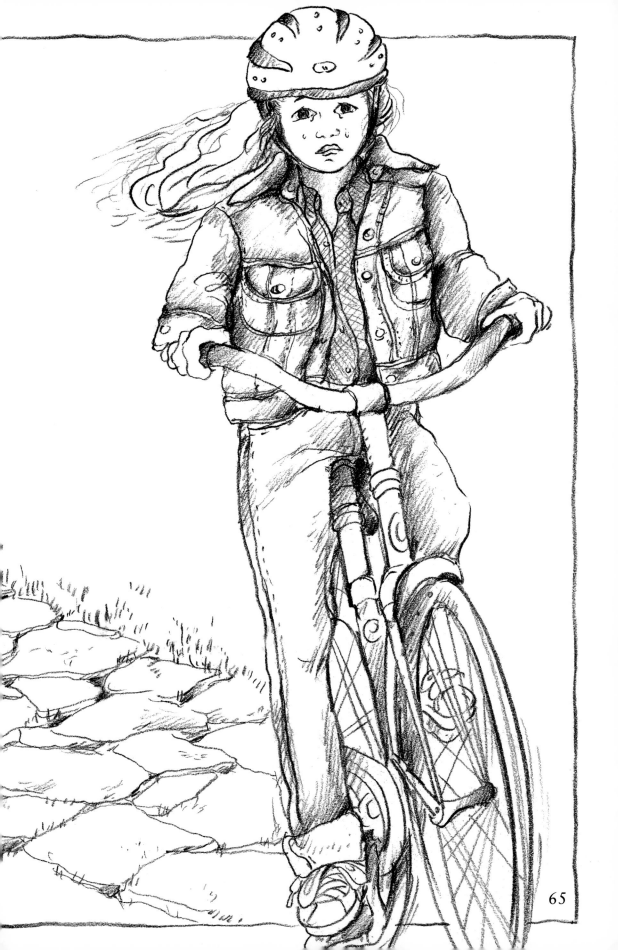

"Hi!" said Erin's mom. "Did you have a nice time playing with Brandi?"

"It was okay," Erin said. Erin wanted to cry.

Erin's Mom knew something was wrong. "You always have so much fun with Brandi," Erin's mom said. "Did you have fun today?"

"I don't know," said Erin.

Erin's mom knew that Erin was unhappy. But she didn't know why.

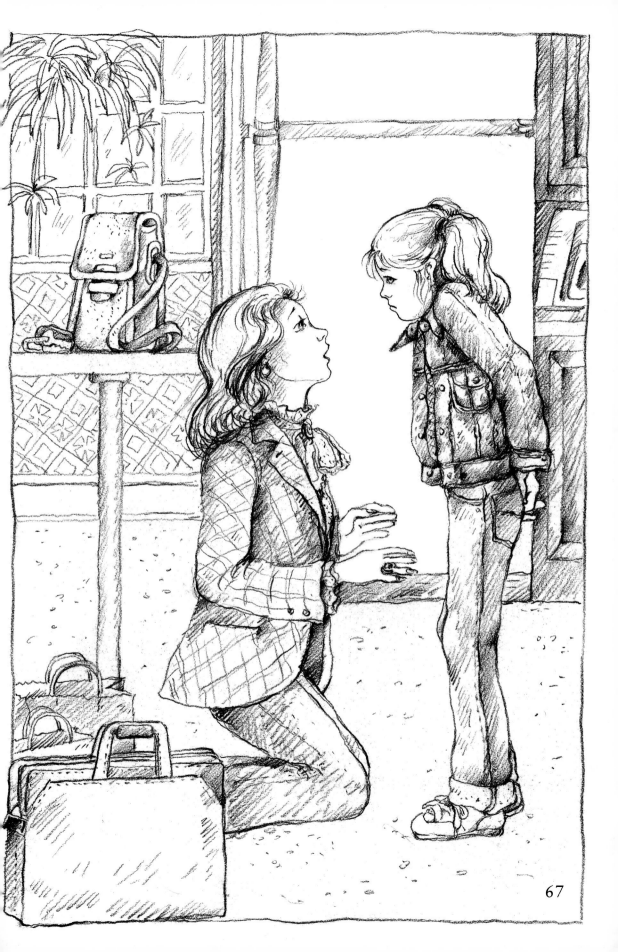

In the middle of the night, something woke Erin up. She felt cold. Her pajamas were wet. Her bed was wet.

"Oh, no!" she thought. "I did it *again!* I wet when I was sleeping *again!*"

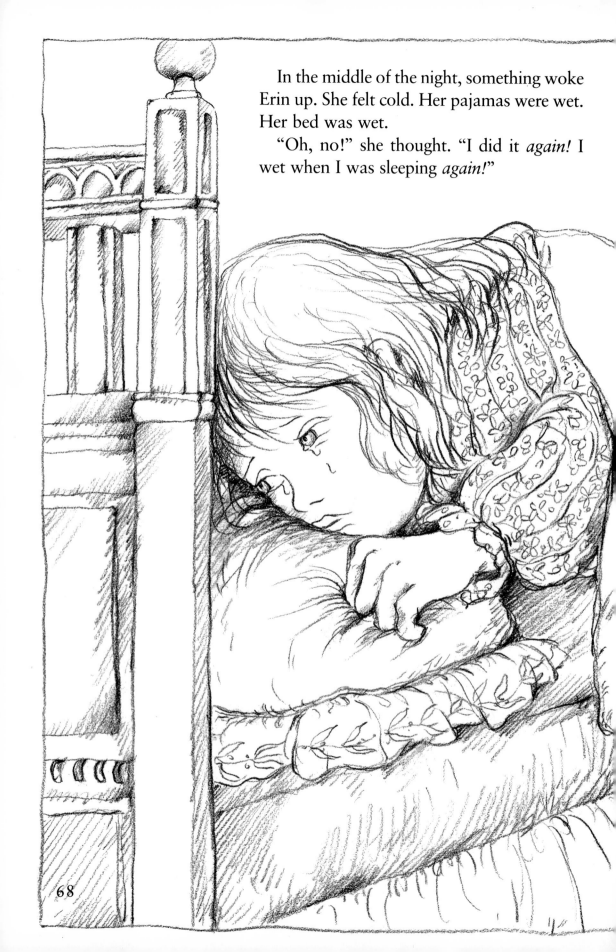

Erin began to cry. "That's why I couldn't stay overnight at Brandi's house," Erin cried. "Because I was afraid I would wet when I was sleeping! Brandi would find out that I wet. What if she told the other kids in our class? They would think I was a big baby!"

Erin hated the way she felt. She hated the feeling of cold, wet pajamas. She hated the feeling of a cold, wet bed. She hated being afraid to sleep over at Brandi's house. She hated worrying about what other kids would think.

Erin was sad. She wanted to be dry all night so much! She cried and cried and cried and cried and cried.

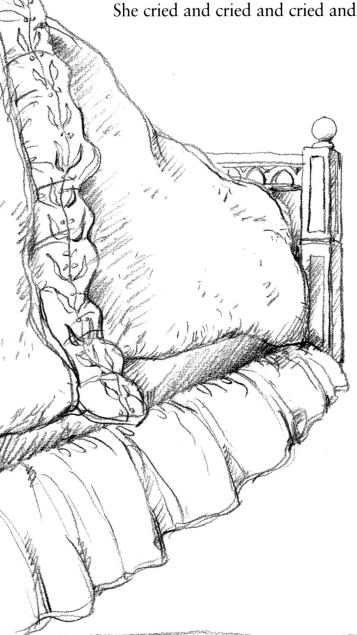

Erin's mom heard her crying. When she came into Erin's room she knew right away what was wrong.

"Don't cry, Erin," she said. "It's not your fault that you wet when you're sleeping. I don't care about a silly old wet bed. All I care about is *you!* I love you very, very much. You're always so nice to people. You do so many things really well. Wetting when you're sleeping isn't a big

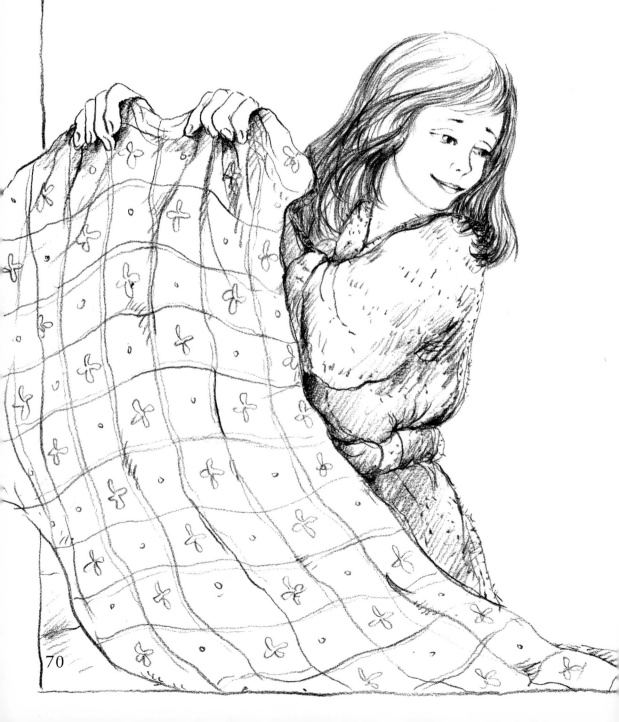

thing at all. It's nothing to be ashamed of. Lots of kids do it. Sooner or later they always stop."

"But I want to stop *now*," said Erin. "I don't want to wet when I'm sleeping anymore. I want to *do* something about it!"

"I know what you can do," said Erin's mom. "You're very smart and you like to read. Today I got a new book for you. It'll tell you the easy things you can do to stop wetting when you're sleeping. I'll give it to you as a present tomorrow. You're going to have fun reading it. You'll be able to do the things you need to do all by yourself."

"Great," said Erin. "I like reading books and finding out new things!"

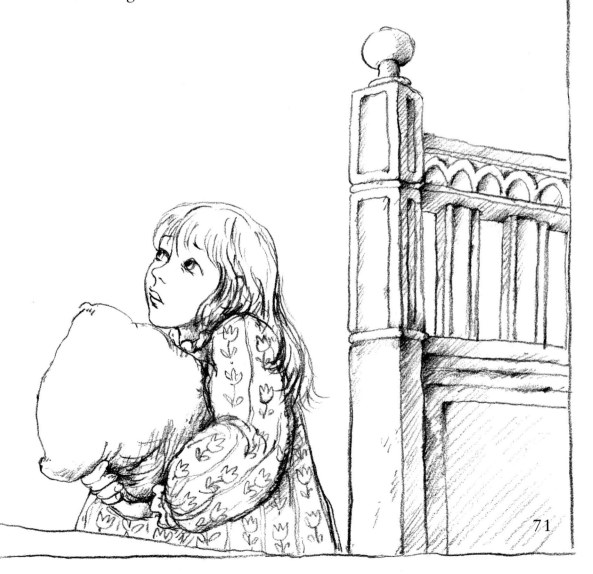

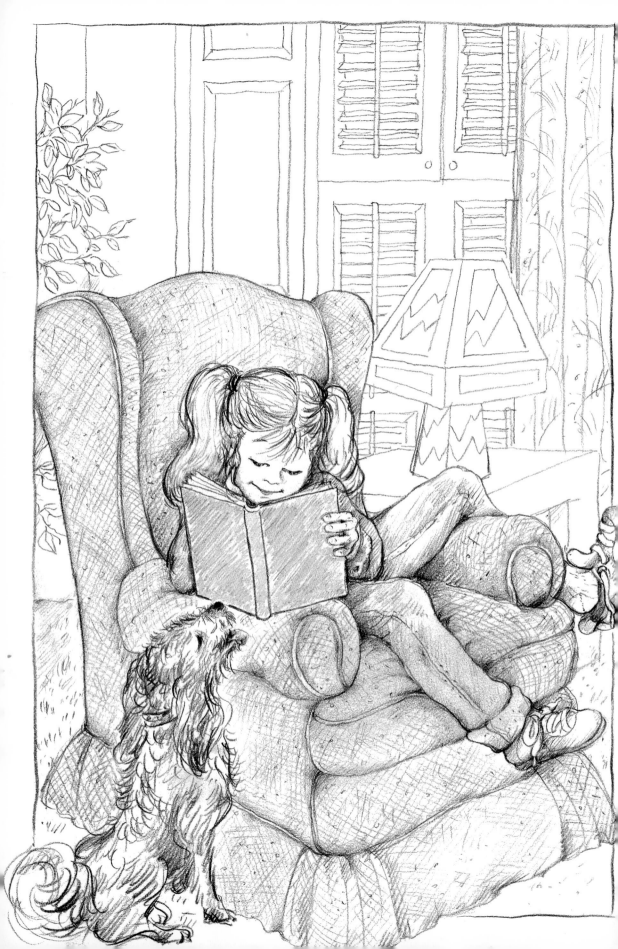

The next day, Erin read her new book. The name of her book was *Dry All Night*. She liked reading it. It told her what she needed to do to be dry all night. The things it told her to do were easy and looked like fun. She could do them all by herself.

The book was a story about a boy named Christopher . . .

Christopher was really good at karate. He could do the most amazing jumps and kicks. All the kids thought he was really special. They all wanted to be his friend. He was Master Lee's best student.

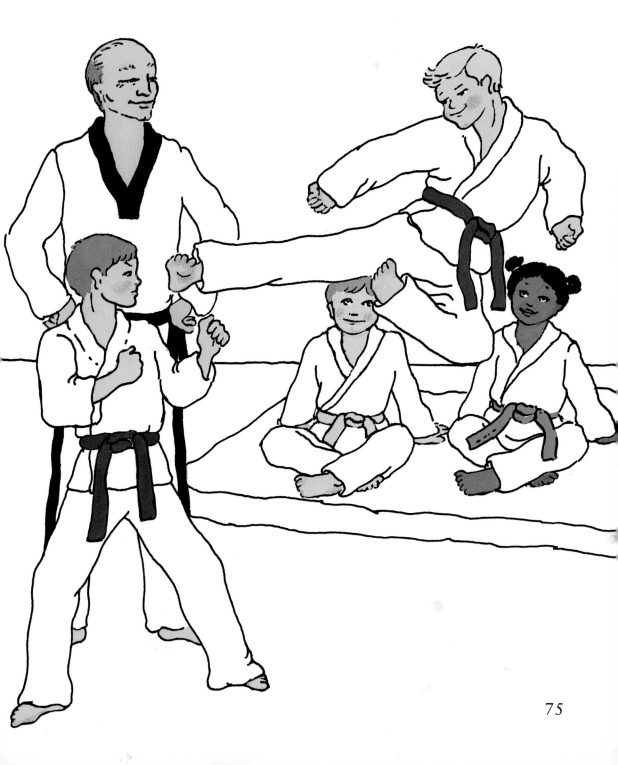

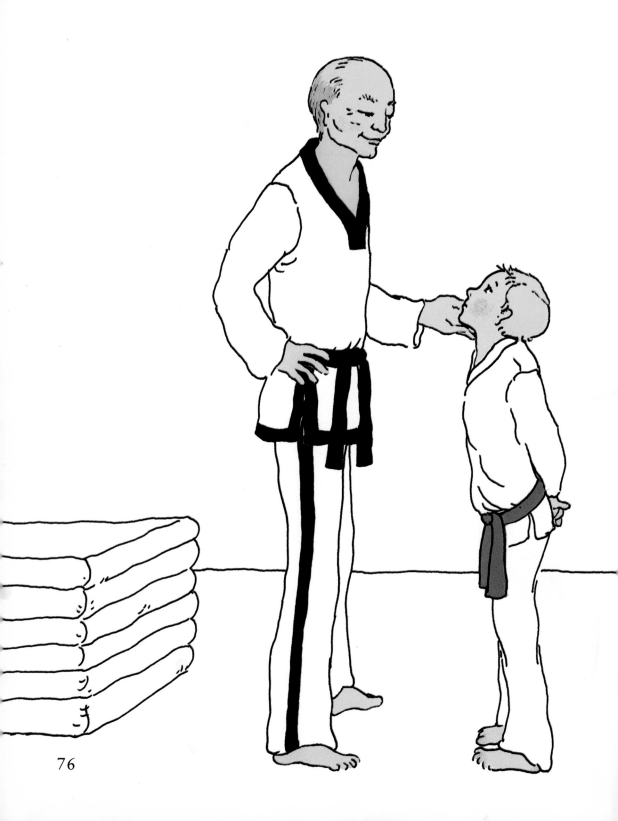

After class, Master Lee said, "Christopher, I want you to come to karate camp this summer. I am asking only my best students. The camp is for older children, but I am certain that you are grown-up enough. It is time for you to learn to use the power of your mind to control all the parts of your body."

Christopher was honored to be asked to come to karate camp. It made him very happy. He wanted to say yes to Master Lee. But he couldn't.

"I *want* to come —" Christopher said. But then he stopped. He didn't know how to tell Master Lee that he couldn't come to karate camp.

Master Lee smiled gently. "Is something wrong, Christopher?"

"No . . ." Christopher said. But there was.

"Good," said Master Lee. "Then it is settled."

Christopher gulped. "But I'll — I'll have to ask when I get home."

"Of course," said Master Lee. "Nothing is more important than respect for parents."

Christopher was all alone in the locker room after his karate class. He was very unhappy. Master Lee was counting on him to come to karate camp. But how could he go?

How could a kid who wet when he was sleeping go to sleep-away camp?

The other kids would find out. Master Lee would find out.

"Oh," said Christopher. "I *hate* wetting when I'm sleeping! I *hate* lying in a wet bed all night long! I want to stop wetting so much! I wish I were dry all night!"

All of a sudden, a camel appeared.

"Did I hear someone say 'dry all night'?" boomed the camel in a deep voice.

Christopher was so surprised. "Who are *you?*" he said.

"My name is Dan. I'm a magic camel. I like to help kids. My name stands for **D**ry **A**ll **N**ight. And that's what I'm here to help you to be: dry all night."

"But I wet and wet and wet," Christopher said. "I can't believe I'll *ever* be dry all night."

"Believe it," Dan said. "Magic camels don't appear in karate-school locker rooms unless they're *very* serious.

"Come on, Christopher," said Dan. "I'll get you over this hump.

"Hop on board. We're going to a special place called —

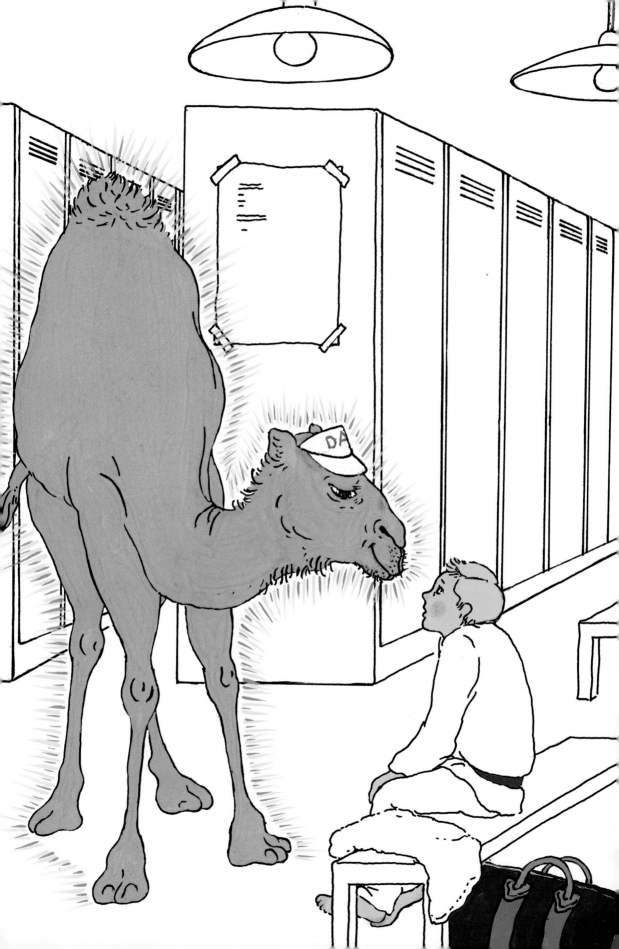

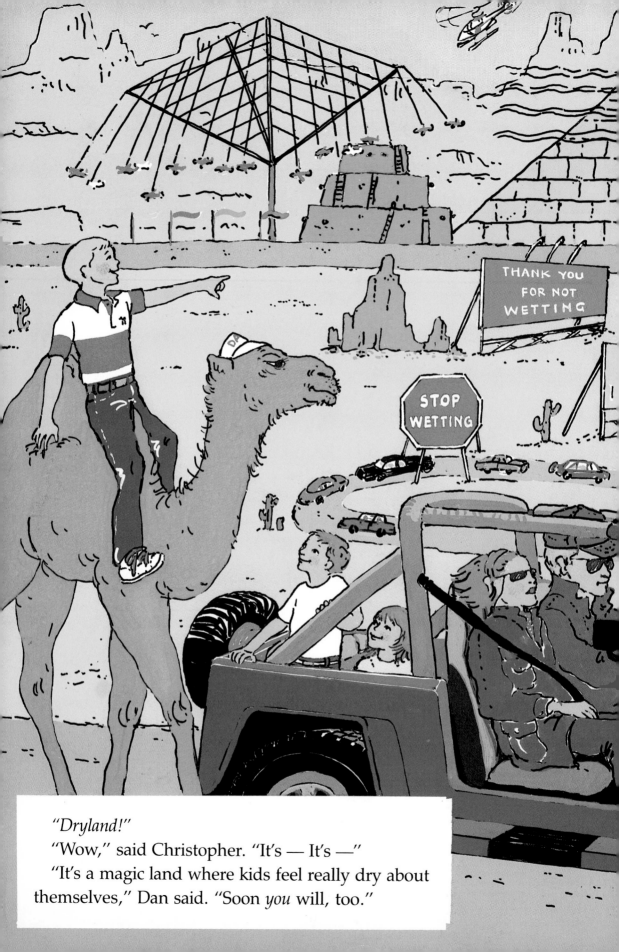

"*Dryland!*"

"Wow," said Christopher. "It's — It's —"

"It's a magic land where kids feel really dry about themselves," Dan said. "Soon *you* will, too."

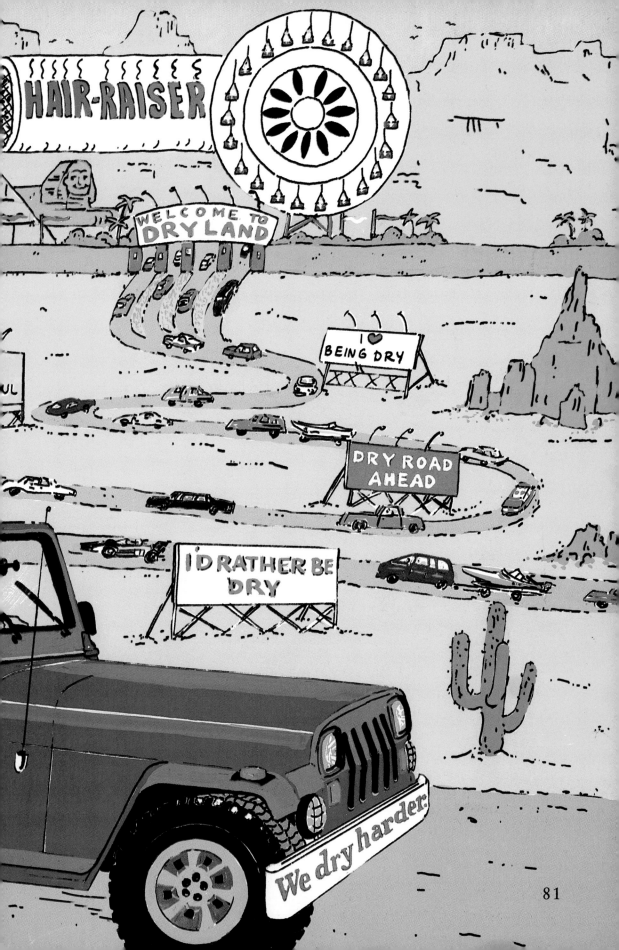

81

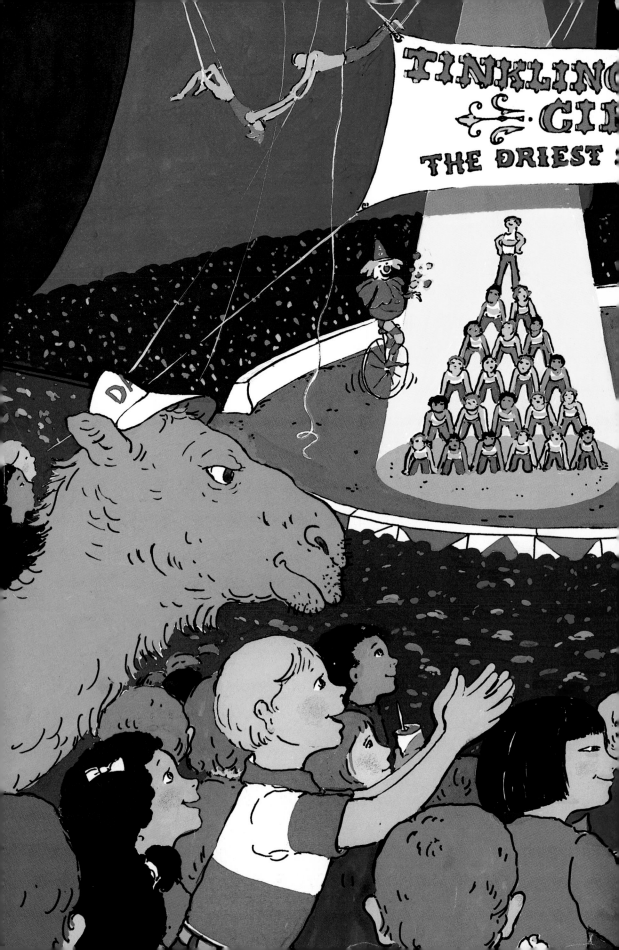

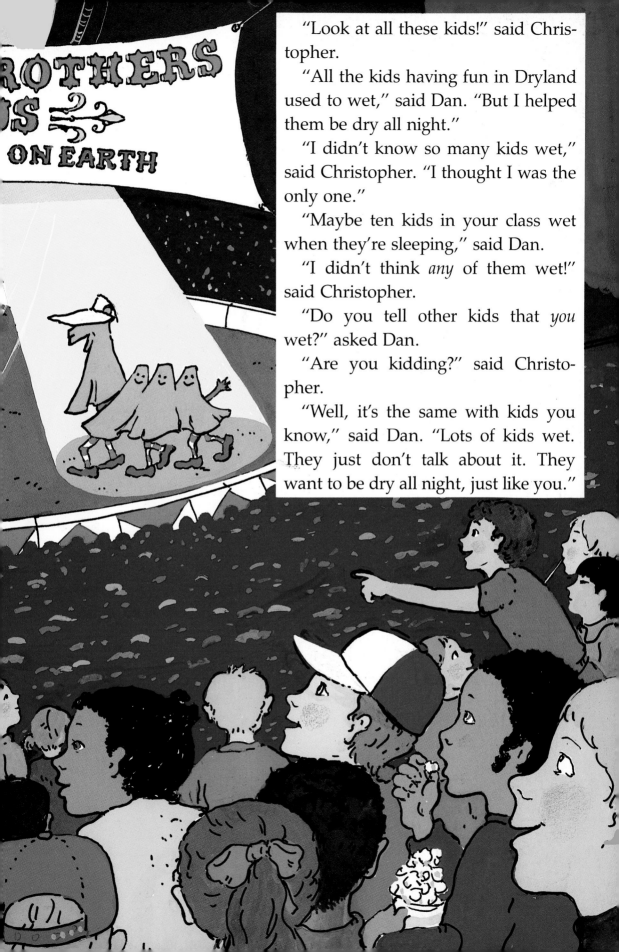

"Look at all these kids!" said Christopher.

"All the kids having fun in Dryland used to wet," said Dan. "But I helped them be dry all night."

"I didn't know so many kids wet," said Christopher. "I thought I was the only one."

"Maybe ten kids in your class wet when they're sleeping," said Dan.

"I didn't think *any* of them wet!" said Christopher.

"Do you tell other kids that *you* wet?" asked Dan.

"Are you kidding?" said Christopher.

"Well, it's the same with kids you know," said Dan. "Lots of kids wet. They just don't talk about it. They want to be dry all night, just like you."

"Knowing what's going on inside you will help you be dry all night," said Dan.

"Inside your belly, there's a bladder. In your bladder there's urine. Urine is mostly water. Part of what you drink becomes urine, because your body doesn't need it anymore. Your bladder holds the urine till you're ready to go to the bathroom.

"Your bladder is a lot like a fire truck," said Dan. "Fire fighters fill up their fire truck with water. Fire trucks can hold lots of water inside.

"When the fire fighters go to a fire and there's no fire hydrant, they can shoot the water that's inside their truck at the fire to put the fire out.

"When the fire fighters want the water inside their truck to go out, it goes out. When they don't want the water to go out, it doesn't go out. The water stays inside the fire truck as long as they want it to stay inside.

"It's the same with your bladder. When you want the urine inside your bladder to go out, it goes out. Up till now, sometimes when you were sleeping the urine inside your bladder went out by accident.

"But you're going to change that, all by yourself. When you don't want the urine inside your bladder to go out, it won't go out.

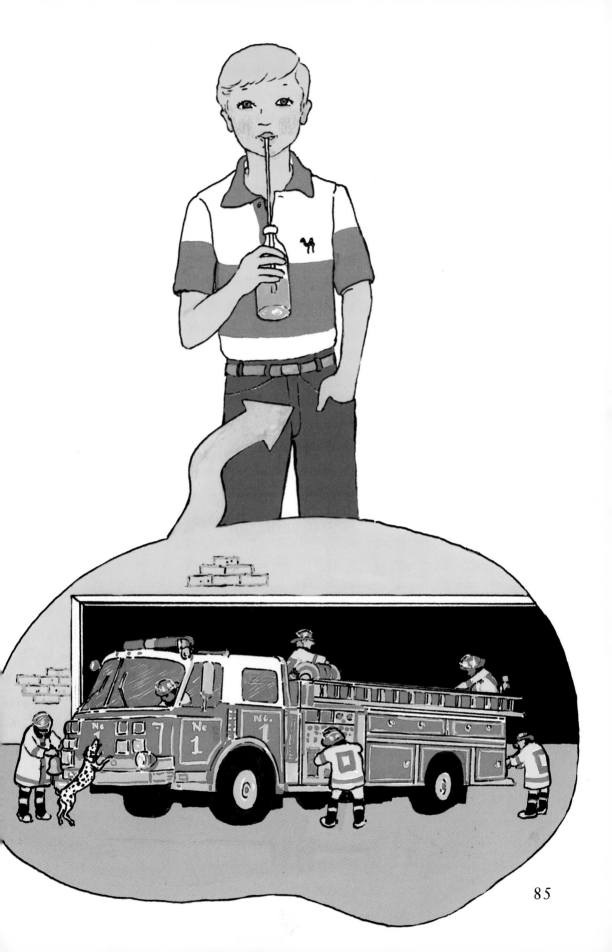

"Inside your head there's a brain," said Dan. "You use your brain to think with. Your brain tells all the parts of your body what to do. Do you know what a fire chief is?"

"Sure," said Christopher. "The fire chief is the boss over all the fire fighters. If the fire chief tells his fire truck to shoot water out, the water shoots out. If the fire chief tells his fire truck not to shoot water out, the water doesn't shoot out."

"Your brain is like the fire chief," said Dan. "Just the way the fire chief is the boss over his fire truck, your brain is the boss over your bladder."

"So I can be the boss over my bladder by using my brain!" said Christopher. "I'll be just like a fire chief!"

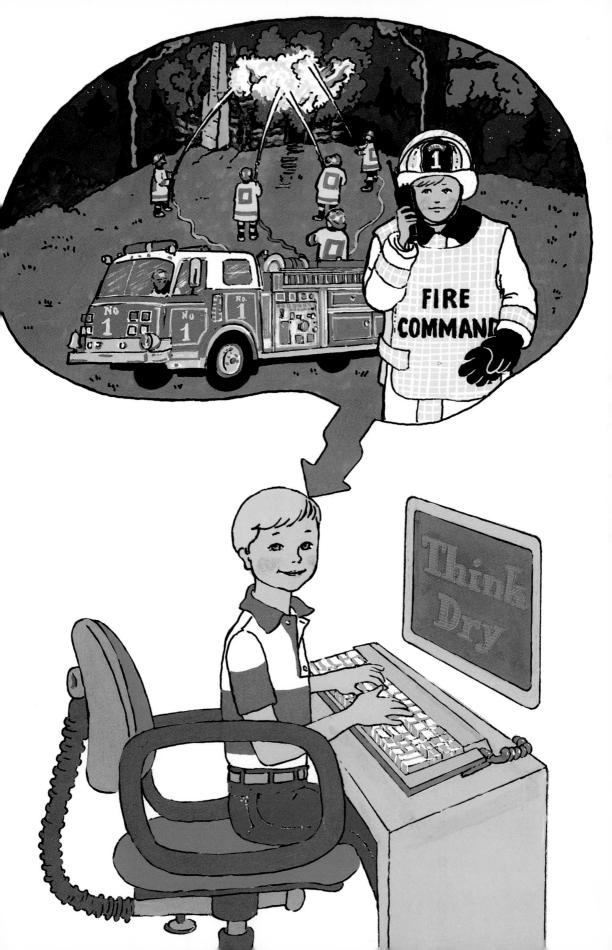

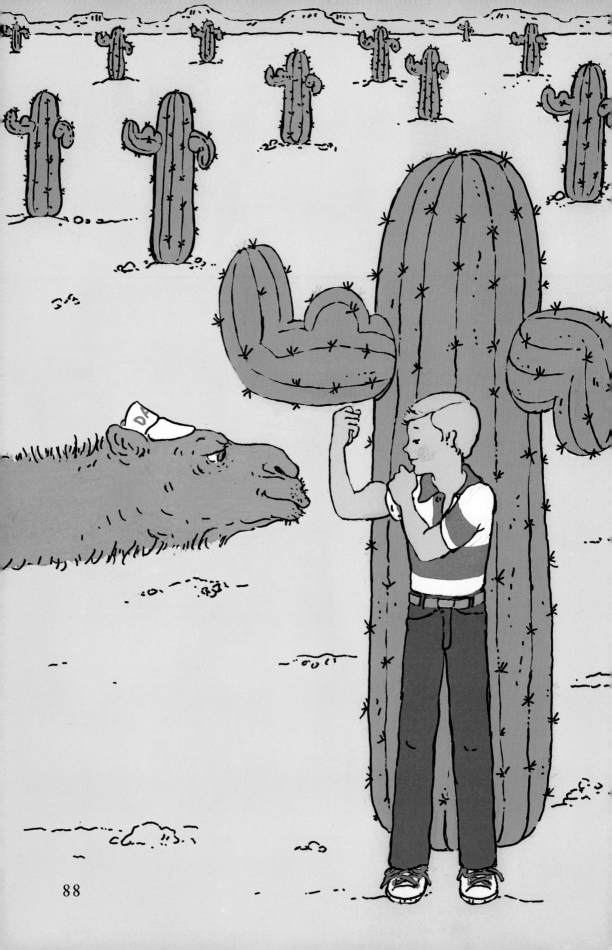

"Your bladder is a *muscle*," said Dan.

"Like the muscle I make with my arm?" asked Christopher.

"Right," said Dan. "How do you make your arm muscle do what you want?"

"I guess I just *think* about it," said Christopher. Then Christopher had an idea: "I know!" he said. "I use my brain to be the boss over my arm muscle!"

"You can use your brain to be the boss over all your muscles," said Dan.

"There are muscles in your legs. By being the boss over the muscles in your legs, you can run.

"There are muscles in your mouth. By being the boss over the muscles in your mouth, you can talk.

"You can wink and smile and scrunch up your nose and wiggle your toes whenever you want to, because you're the boss over all your muscles.

"And you can be the boss over your bladder, too, because your bladder is a muscle."

"But I wet when I'm *sleeping*," said Christopher. "How can I use my brain to be the boss over my bladder muscle when I'm fast asleep?"

"Your brain is awake *all* the time, even when you're sleeping," said Dan.

"If you're too hot when you're sleeping, your brain tells the muscles in your legs to kick off the blankets.

"If you're too close to the edge of the bed when you're sleeping, your brain tells your muscles to move you so you won't fall out of bed.

"If you hear a loud noise when you're sleeping, your brain tells you to wake up really fast.

"From now on, if your bladder muscle gets all filled up with urine when you're sleeping, it can just stay full, all night long, without any urine going out.

"But if your bladder muscle feels like maybe it won't be able to hold the urine all night long, your brain is going to tell you to wake up really fast."

"Great," said Christopher. "When my brain wakes me up, I'll be able to go to the bathroom and put the urine in the toilet, where I want it to go."

"Good," said Dan. "There's a special ride here in Dryland where I can show you how you're going to be the boss over your bladder muscle. Would you like to go on it?"

"I sure would!" said Chris.

"Then let's go!" said Dan.

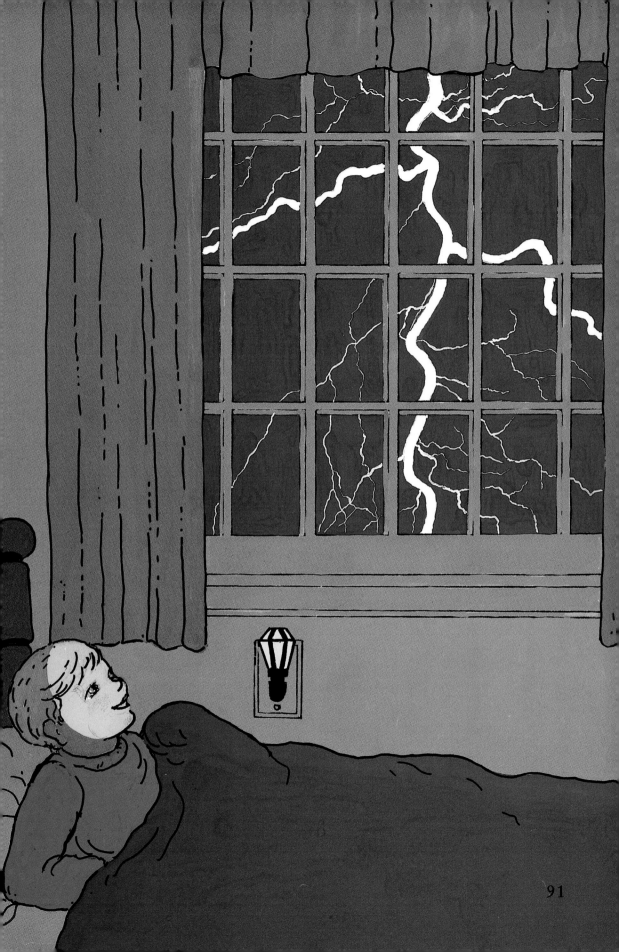

"Here we are at the Dryland Fire Chief Ride," said Dan.

"Wow!" said Christopher.

"First you'll go upstairs in the fire house," Dan said. "You'll get into the fire chief's bed and make believe you're sleeping. Then the fire bell will ring really, really loud. When the bell rings, it'll wake you right up. You'll jump out of bed and put on your fire chief suit.

"Then you'll slide down the pole like a fire chief. You'll get into your fire truck and drive very fast to the fire. Then you'll make the truck shoot water at the fire, the way a fire chief does."

"This ride is fun," said Christopher. "Just the way I'm the boss over my truck on the Fire Chief Ride, I'm going to be the boss over my bladder muscle when I'm sleeping.

"If my bladder muscle gets all filled up with urine, the full feeling can wake me right up, just like a fire bell ringing really, really loud. Then I'll walk into the bathroom and put the urine in the toilet."

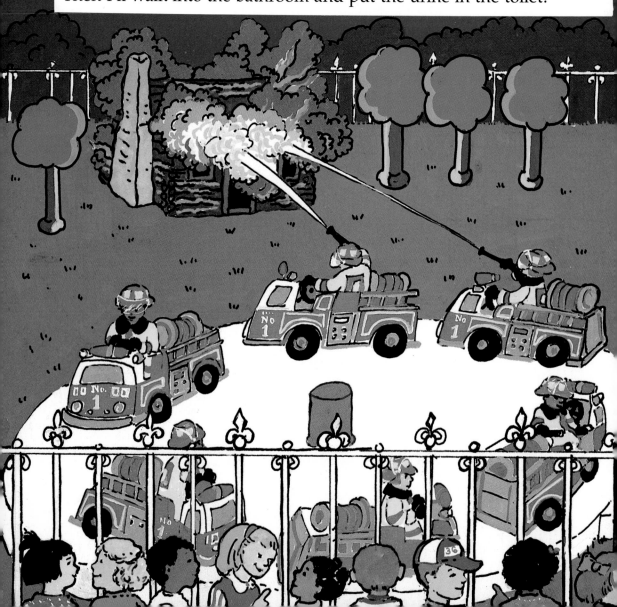

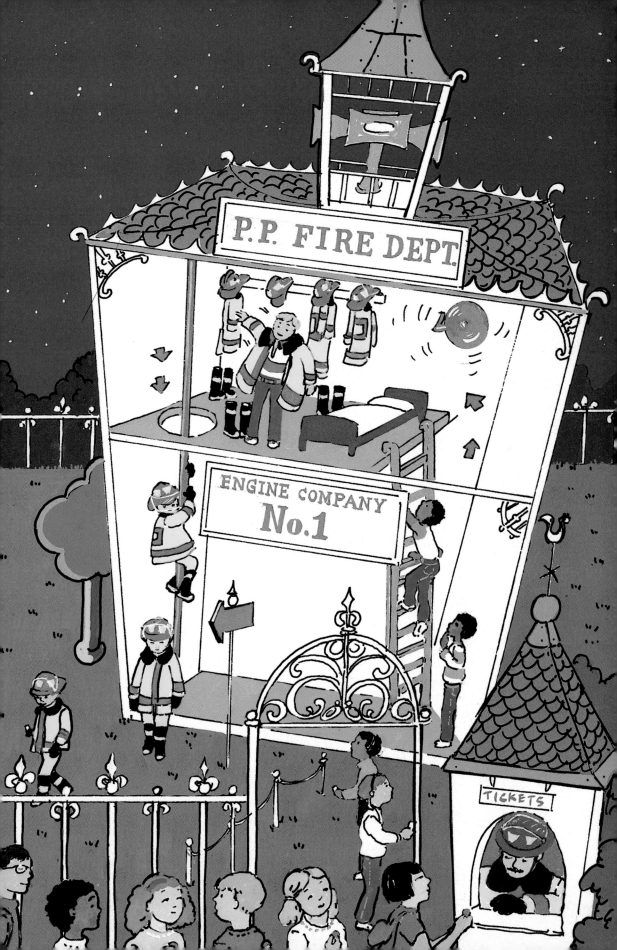

"Every day, you're going to practice being the boss over your bladder muscle by making believe that you're a fire chief being the boss over your fire truck," said Dan.

"Every day, you're going to see a picture in your mind of yourself having fun being a fire chief. It'll look like a TV picture, right inside your head."

"Hey," said Christopher. "That's just like what Master Lee taught me! He taught me to make my jumps and kicks better by seeing a picture inside my head of myself doing jumps and kicks. He taught me that I can be the boss over all the muscles in my body by seeing pictures inside my head."

"Come on," said Dan. "Let's go to another ride in Dryland, where I can show you how easy it's going to be for you to see pictures inside your head of you being the boss over your bladder muscle."

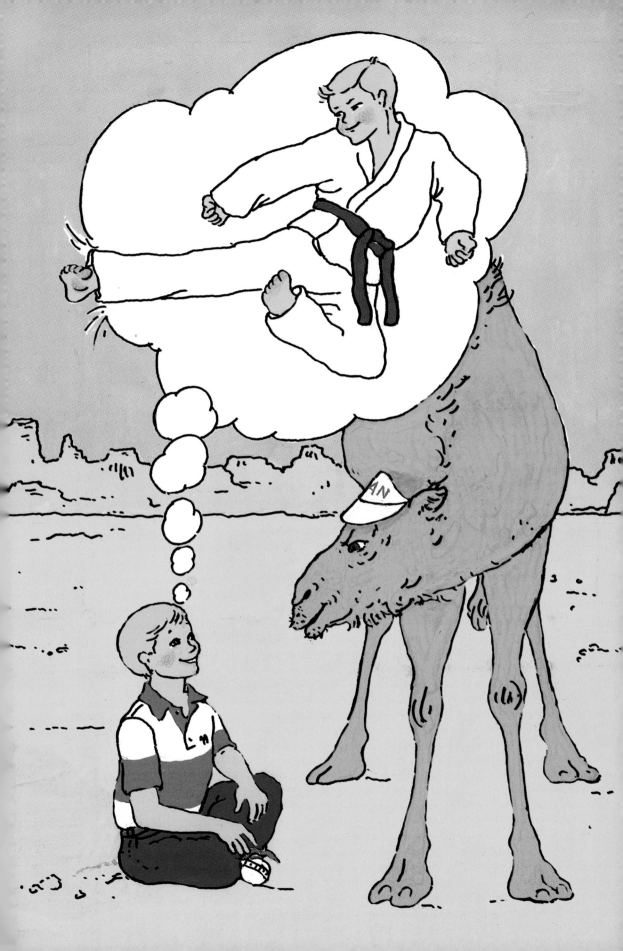

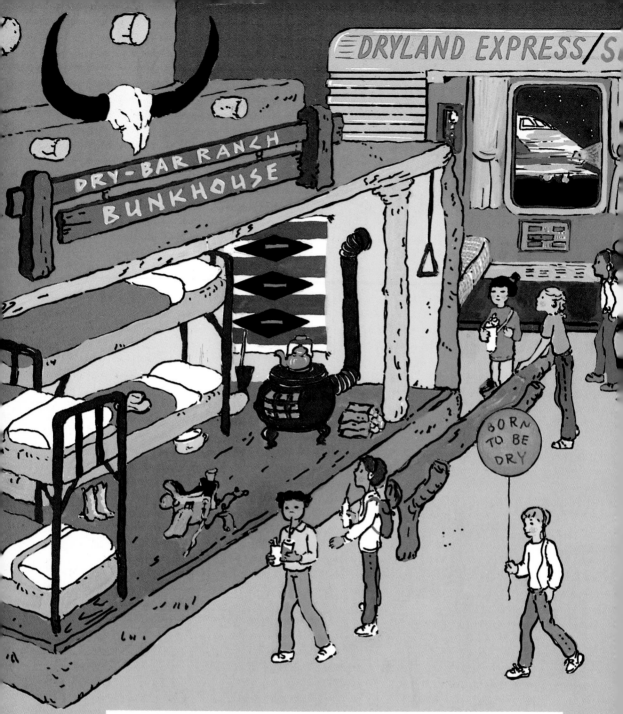

"Wow," said Christopher. "Where are we now?"

"This is the Dryland Super Bed-a-Rama," said Dan. "It's a ride with lots of different places where kids can sleep. I want you to sit on your favorite bed and see pictures inside your head of you being the boss over your bladder muscle."

"I want to sit on the President's bed," said Christopher.

"Okay," said Dan. "Go for it!"

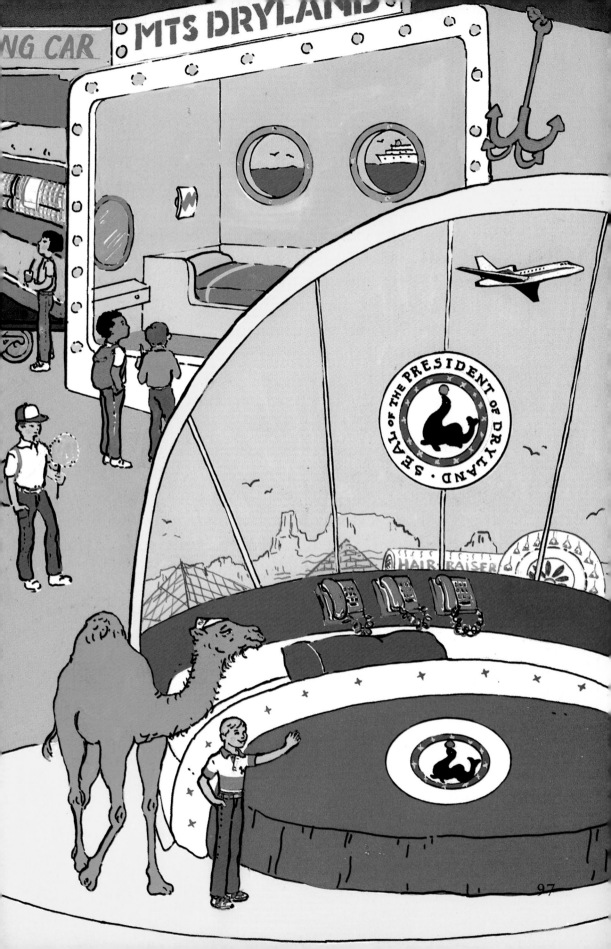

"First I want you to see a picture inside your head of yourself on the Fire Chief Ride," said Dan. "See yourself sleeping in the fire chief's bed. If your fire truck is all filled up with water, it can just stay full, without any water coming out.

"But sometimes the fire bell rings, really, really loud. The bell is so loud that it wakes you up very fast. You jump out of bed. You get into your truck and drive to the fire and shoot all the water at it."

"I see the picture!" said Christopher. "It's easy for me to see it. It looks like a TV picture. I can hear the fire bell ringing. I see myself in a suit and a hat, being a fire chief. I see myself having lots of fun on the Fire Chief Ride, being the boss over my fire truck."

"Your bladder muscle is like a fire truck that can get all filled up with water," said Dan. "Tell yourself that if your bladder muscle gets all filled up with urine when you're sleeping, it can just stay full, all night long, without any urine going out. Or, the full feeling will wake you up right away, just like a fire bell ringing really, really loud.

"Tell yourself that as soon as you wake up, you're going to walk to the bathroom and put the urine in the toilet, where you want it to go.

"When you're putting the urine in the toilet, I think you're going to feel really good, because you're the boss over your bladder muscle, just like the fire chief is the boss over his fire truck."

"Soon urine will go out of my bladder only when I'm wide-awake," said Christopher. "I'll be dry all night!"

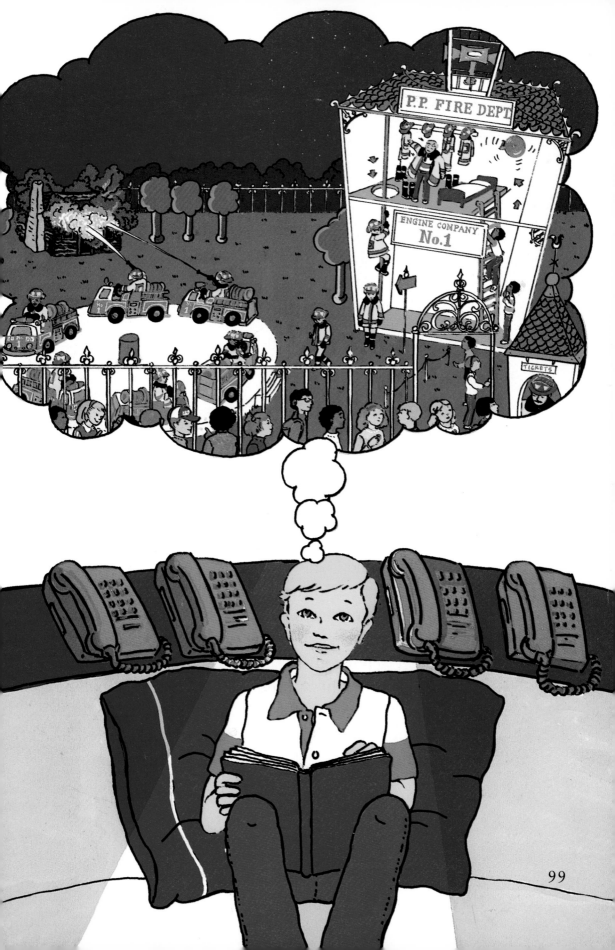

"Now I want you to see another picture inside your head," said Dan. "I want you to see a picture of yourself getting out of bed because the feeling of your bladder muscle being all filled up with urine was like a fire bell ringing really, really loud and woke you right up so you can walk to the bathroom.

"Make believe you're waking up," said Dan. "When you wake up I think you're going to feel really good because your pajamas are soft and dry.

"Make believe that you sit up in your bed as soon as you wake up. It's nice and quiet in the middle of the night. You can see that there's one little light on in your room.

"You're going to get out of bed so you can put the urine in the toilet, where you want it to go. Make believe that you feel your feet touch the floor when you get out of bed.

"From now on, every afternoon, and every night before you go to sleep, I want you to sit on your bed and have fun seeing these pictures inside your head, one after another, just like on TV," said Dan.

"When you see these pictures of you being the boss over your bladder muscle, I want you to tell yourself that you're only going to urinate when you're wide-awake.

"I want you to tell your bladder muscle that if it gets all filled up with urine when you're sleeping, it can just stay full, all night long, without any urine going out. Or, the full feeling will be like a fire bell ringing really, really loud, waking you right up.

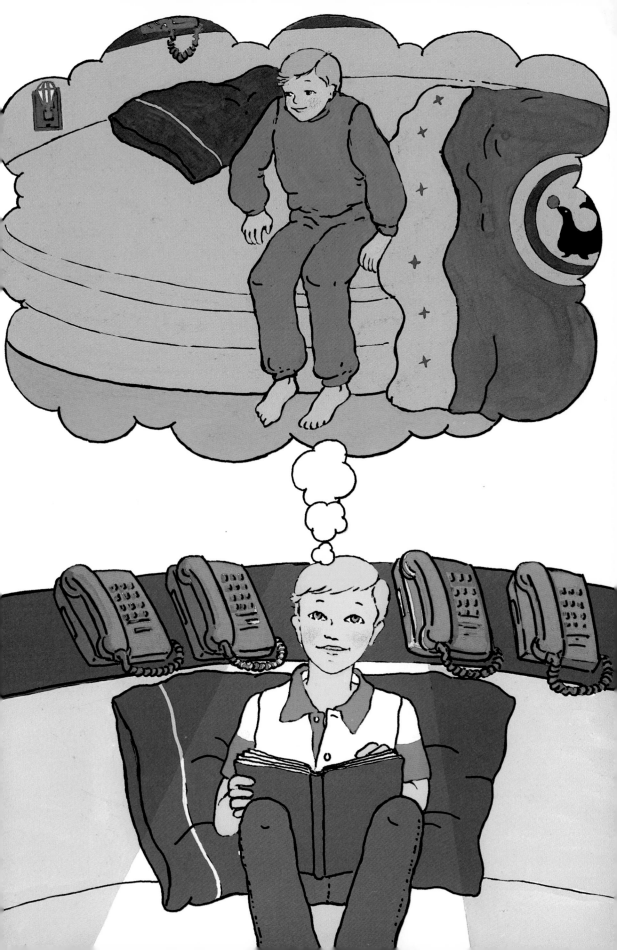

"Now I want you to see another picture inside your head," said Dan. "I want you to see a picture of yourself in the bathroom, urinating into the toilet.

"Make believe that you woke right up because your bladder muscle felt like it was all filled up with urine," said Dan. "Make believe that you got out of bed and walked into the bathroom. You can see that there's one little light on in the bathroom.

"Make believe you're putting the urine in the toilet, where you want it to go. You can hear the sound of the urine going into the toilet. You can even hear the toilet go *whoosh* when you flush it!

"You feel really good about putting the urine in the toilet, because you're the boss over your bladder muscle, just like the fire chief is the boss over his fire truck.

"And you know that as soon as you get back into your bed, you're going to fall asleep right away."

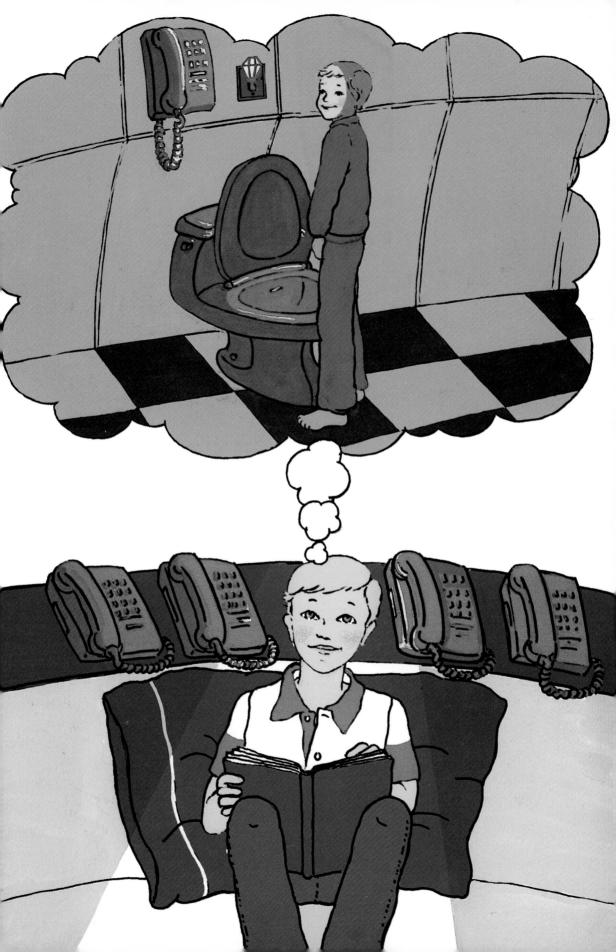

"Now I want you to see another picture inside your head," said Dan. "I want you to see a picture of yourself sleeping in a nice dry bed.

"When you see this picture, I want you to tell yourself that soon you're going to be able to sleep all night long, every night, without any urine going out of your bladder muscle."

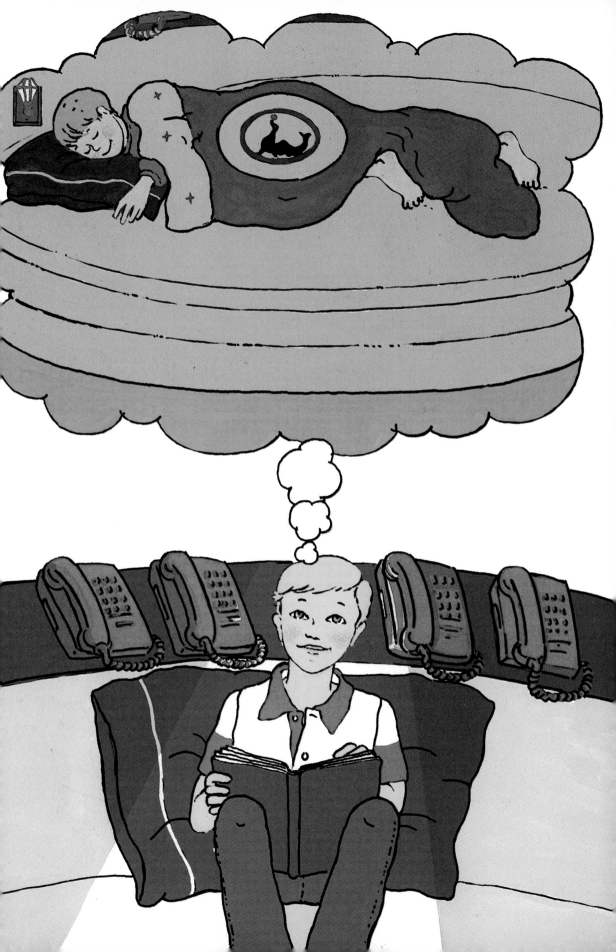

"Now I want you to see another picture inside your head," said Dan. "I want you to see a picture of yourself waking up in the morning after you were dry all night.

"Make believe you didn't wet when you were sleeping," said Dan. "Make believe it's daytime in your room. Make believe you're touching your sheets. They feel nice and dry. Make believe you're touching your blanket, and it feels nice and dry. Now make believe you're touching your pajamas. They feel nice and dry, too.

"Make believe that you feel really, really good because you were the boss over your bladder muscle when you were sleeping.

"Now you've learned how to see the pictures inside your head," said Dan.

"It was so easy!" said Christopher. "Seeing the pictures inside my head was fun. I feel really good now!"

"That's great," said Dan. "Now, let's go to the Drylab and have a look at some good old H_2O."

"What's H_2O?" asked Christopher.

"You already know what it is," said Dan. "Come on — I'll show you.

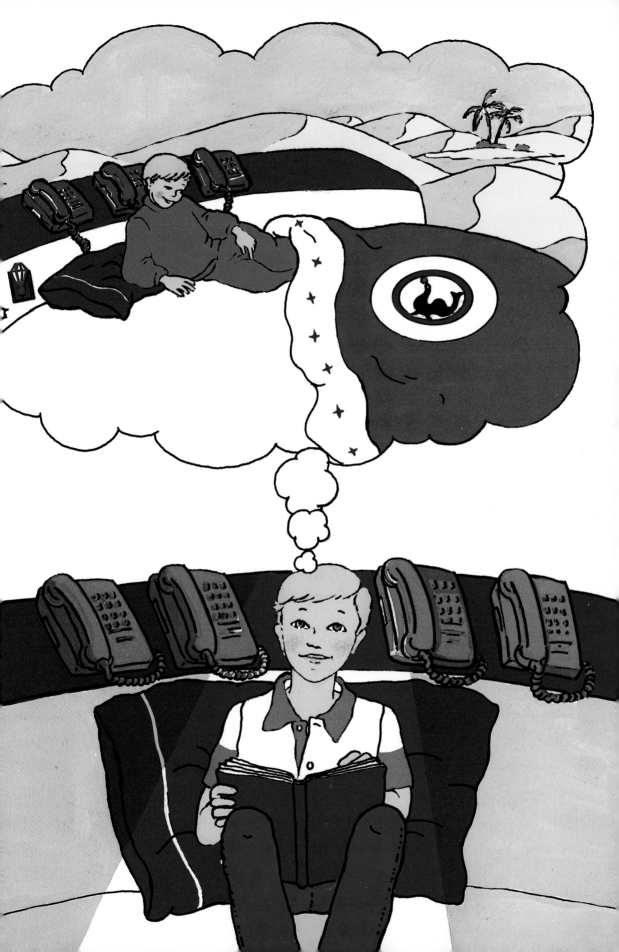

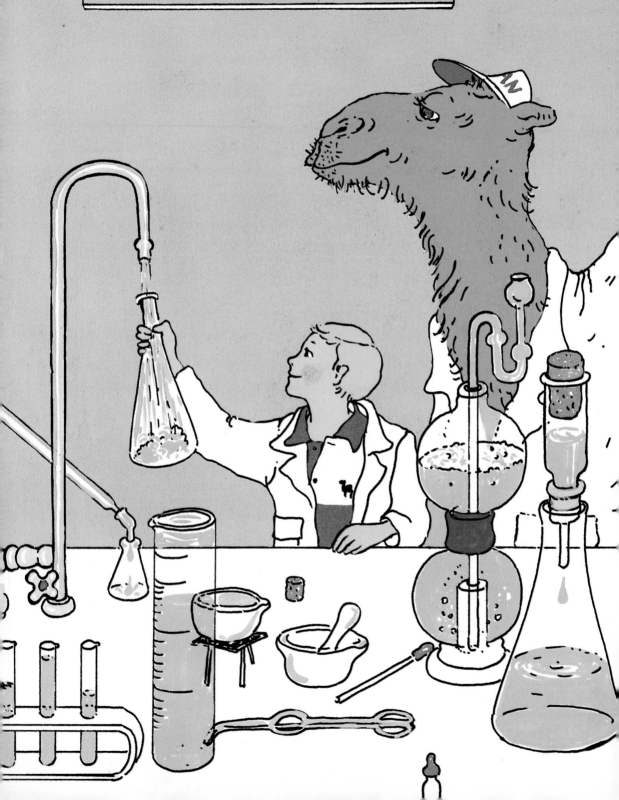

"What's that clear, wet stuff that comes out of the faucets in your house?" asked Dan.

"You mean . . . water?" said Christopher.

"I mean a super-chemical called H_2O!" said Dan.

"H_2O?" said Christopher. "I thought it was just plain water."

"It *is* just plain water," said Dan. "But just plain water is incredible. Because it's around so much, we forget it's so special. But water is really an amazing chemical that scientists call H_2O.

"Water has the power to do lots and lots of things. If you dip a brush in it and touch it to the colors in a paint set, you can make a picture with water. If you fill a bathtub with it, you can sail a toy boat in water. If you put some in a pot, you can cook food in water.

"And one of the things water can do is help you stop wetting when you're asleep.

"I want you to drink lots of water every day. Drinking plenty of powerful H_2O all day will help you be dry all night.

"H$_2$O has the power to make lots of things happen," said Dan. "H$_2$O makes trees and plants grow. Fruits and vegetables come from trees and plants. So water even helps make the food you eat."

"Wow," said Christopher. "H$_2$O can do so many things!"

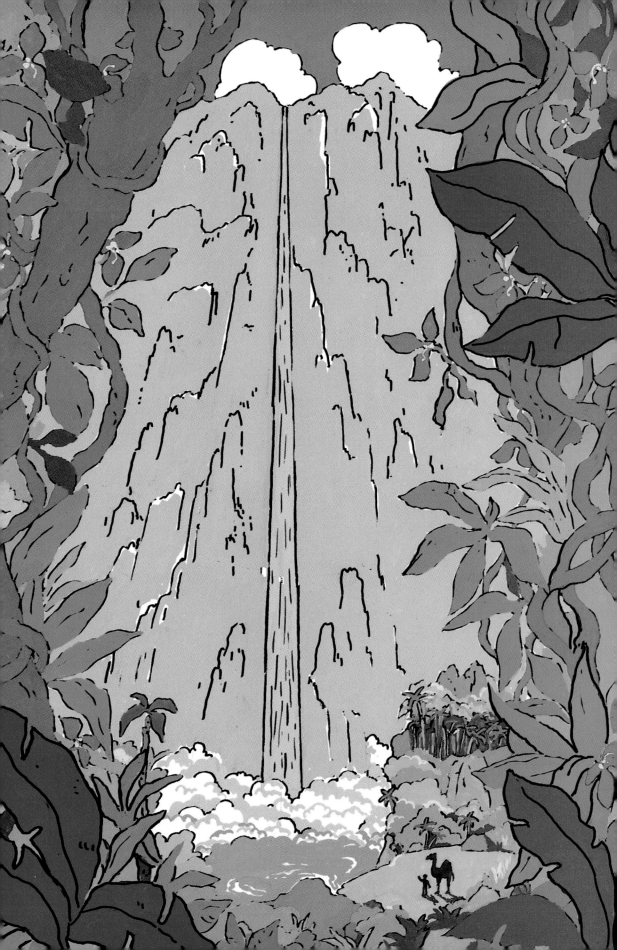

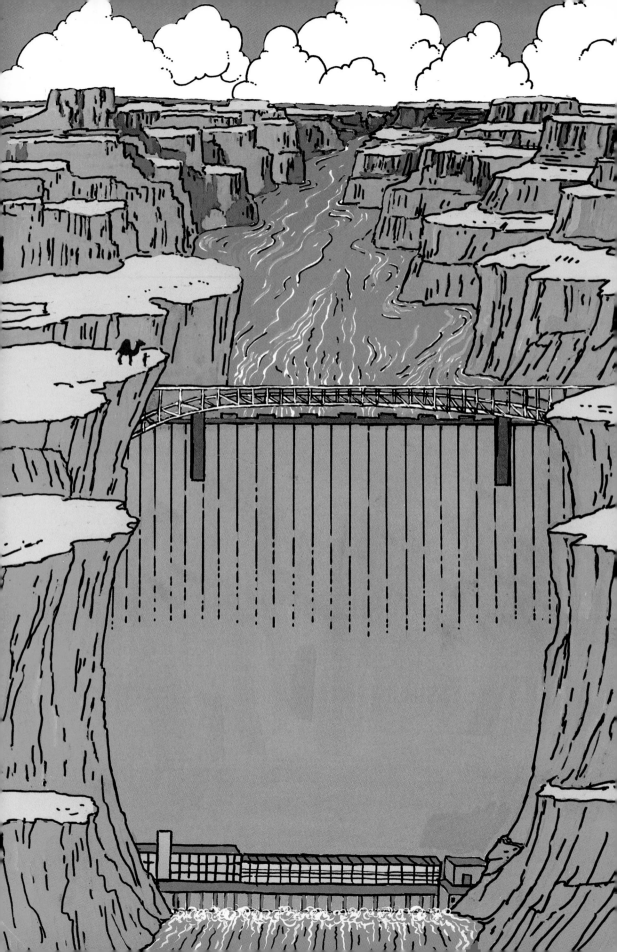

"H$_2$O is very, very powerful," said Dan. "Rivers of water have the power to cut right through the hardest rock to make deep canyons.

"When you build a dam across a river, you can use the power of the water from the river to make electricity, so that people can have lights in their houses, and computers, and TVs.

"And H$_2$O has the power to help you stop wetting when you're asleep. Right now you wet sometimes when you're sleeping, because the bladder muscle inside you is still little.

"But you're getting bigger every day, so your bladder muscle is getting bigger every day, too, especially when you drink lots of water. As soon as your bladder muscle gets just a little bit bigger, you're going to be dry all night."

"I want you to drink plenty of powerful H_2O all day, to help you be dry all night," said Dan. "You'll drink H_2O at school. You'll drink H_2O at friends' houses. You'll drink H_2O at home. You'll drink H_2O everywhere.

"In the daytime, I want you to listen to your bladder muscle. When your bladder muscle tells you it's all filled up with urine, I want you to stop what you're doing and go to the bathroom and urinate into the toilet.

"In the afternoon, right before you sit on your bed and read your *Dry All Night* book and see the pictures inside your head, I want you to drink a great big glass of H_2O.

"After you see the pictures inside your head and finish reading your book, I want you to go into the bathroom and urinate. It'll make you feel good to know that you're the boss over your bladder muscle.

"But after you eat supper, you won't drink anything unless you feel pretty thirsty."

"After supper, I'll think before I drink!" said Christopher.

"Right," laughed Dan.

"Hey, Dan," said Christopher. "What's that big building up on Dryland Mountain?"

"That's the Dry All Knight's Castle," said Dan. "Come on, let's go!"

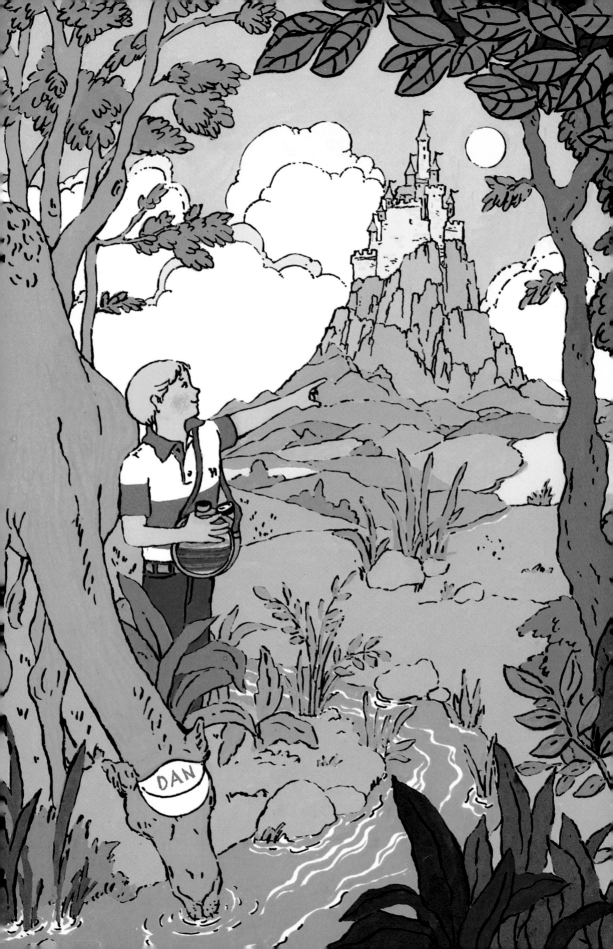

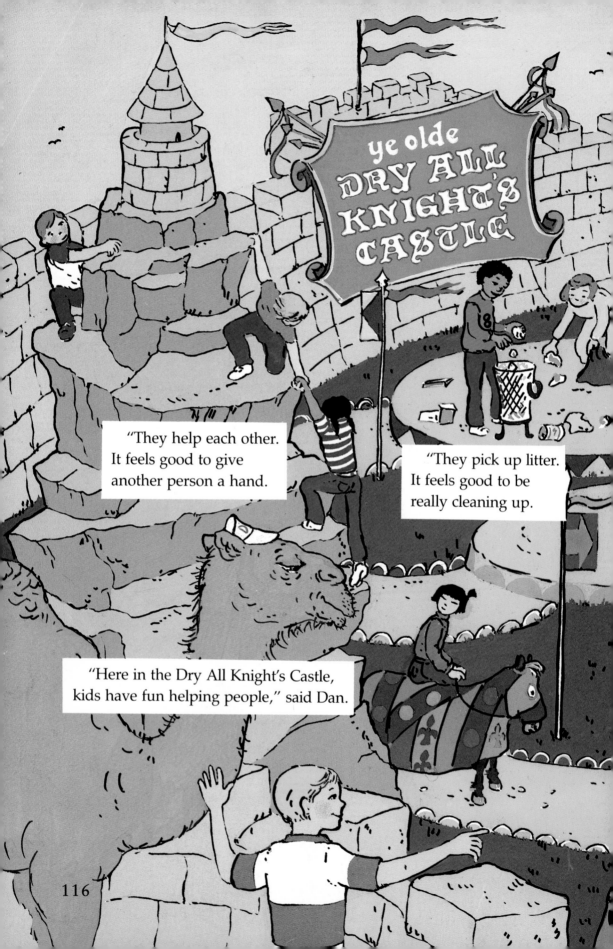

ye olde
DRY ALL
KNIGHT'S
CASTLE

"They help each other.
It feels good to give
another person a hand.

"They pick up litter.
It feels good to be
really cleaning up.

"Here in the Dry All Knight's Castle,
kids have fun helping people," said Dan.

116

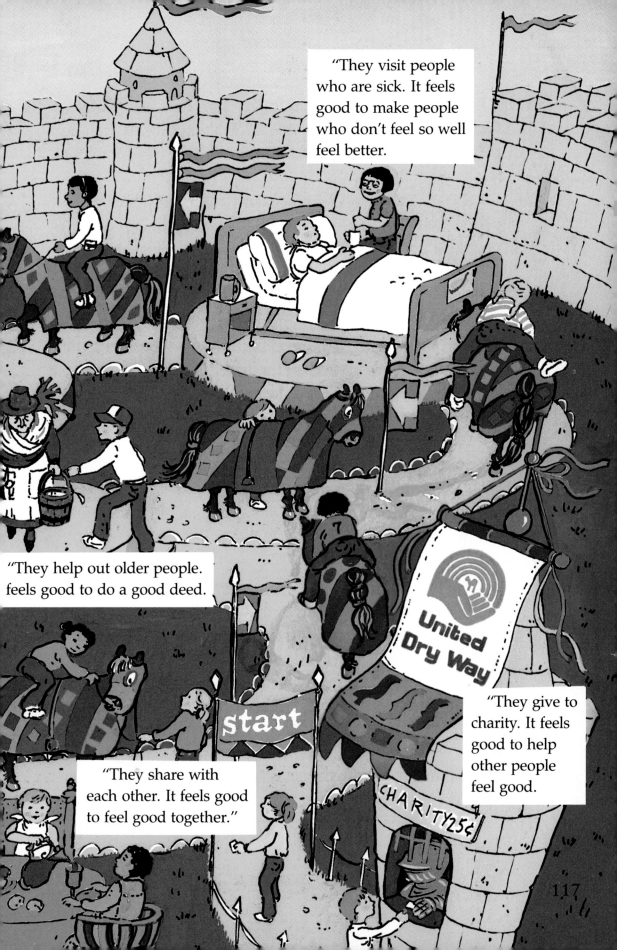

Christopher helped people in the Dry All Knight's Castle. He had lots of fun. "I've always liked helping people," said Christopher. "Helping people makes me feel really good about myself."

"You're going to do more and more nice things for people," said Dan. "Knowing that you're being good to people is going to make you like yourself more and more and more.

"You're growing up really fast, and growing means changing. So lots of new things are going to be happening in your life, things that are going to make you feel better and better about yourself all the time.

"Every day, you're going to become taller and stronger and smarter and more grown-up.

"You're going to like people more and more, and people are going to like you more and more.

"You're hardly ever going to have fights with anybody, because you're going to get along better and better with your family and with other kids and with your teachers and with just about everybody.

"You're going to feel more and more relaxed and happy most of the time, and you aren't going to worry about silly things that really don't matter.

"Hardly anything is going to bother you, because you're going to be having so much fun playing and finding out new things.

"You're going to learn how to do more and more things really well. Knowing that you're getting really good at doing more and more things is going to make you feel better and better about yourself.

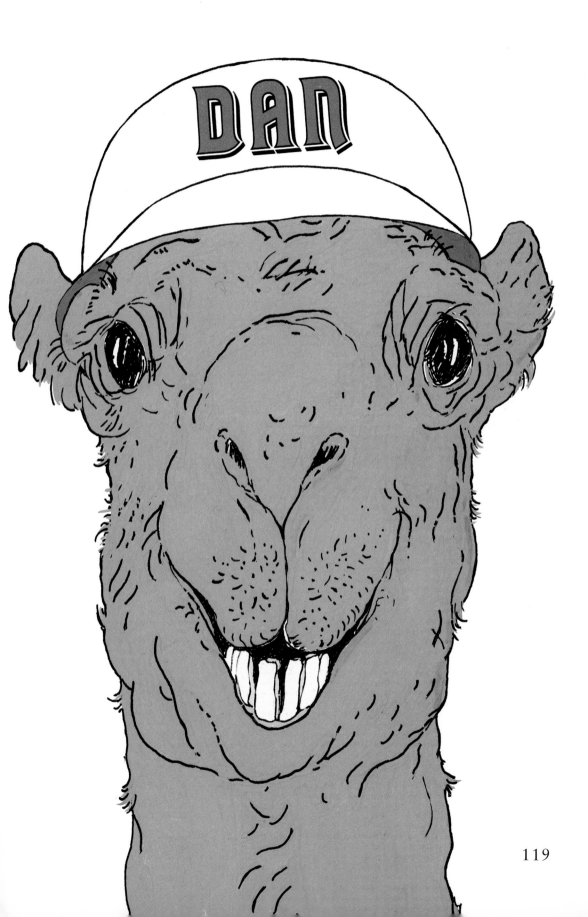

119

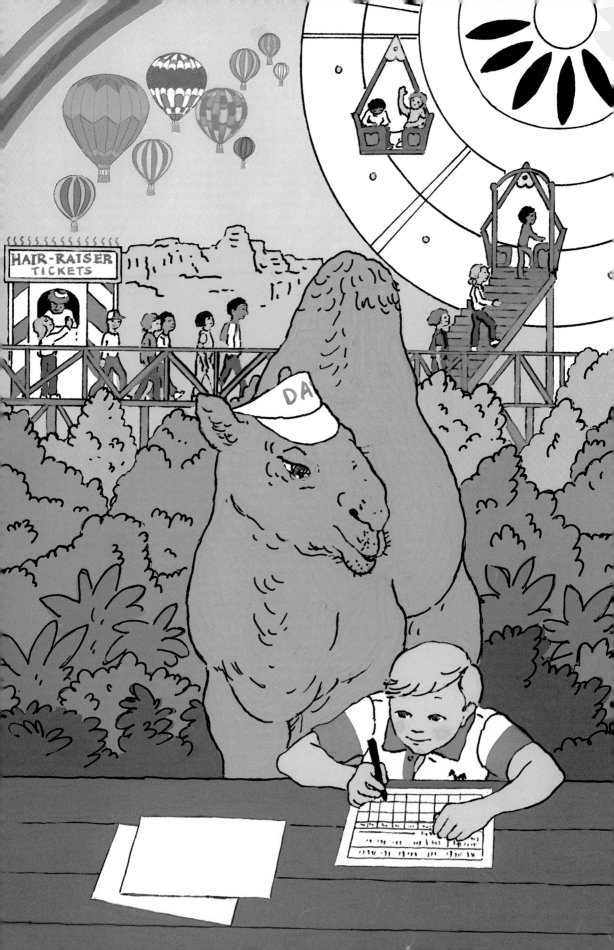

"Now I want you to make a special Dry All Night score-board so you can see how fast you're becoming dry all night," said Dan.

DRY ALL NIGHT				
Week beginning _____ Month / day	I want because :		Sunday	Mon
I was DRY ALL NIGHT last night !				
This afternoon I drank a great big glass of Powerful H_2O			🥛	🥛
Then I sat on my bed and read my DRY ALL NIGHT book			📕📕	📕

"You'll make spaces on your Dry All Night scoreboard for every day of the week," said Dan. "Here's how you'll fill it in:

"At the beginning of every week, I want you to write the most important reason why you want to be dry all night.

"Every afternoon, I want you to drink a great big glass of H_2O. Then I want you to draw a picture of a glass of water on your Dry All Night scoreboard.

"Then I want you to sit on your bed and read your *Dry All Night* book and see the pictures inside your head of you being the boss over your bladder muscle. Then I want you to draw a picture of your *Dry All Night* book on your scoreboard.

"And then I want you to go into the bathroom and urinate into the toilet."

122

SCOREBOARD

DRY ALL NIGHT

week

to go to Karate camp.

:day	Wednesday	Thursday	Friday	Saturday
		🐫	🐫	🐫

"I've got an idea," said Christopher. "When I wake up in the morning and see that I was dry all night, I'm going to draw a picture of *you* on my Dry All Night scoreboard."

"That will make me feel really good," said Dan. "It could take a few days for you to be dry all night. Or it may take a few weeks. Or it might take even more time than that.

"But it won't be long before you'll be drawing *lots* of pictures of me. Because pretty soon, you're going to be dry all night *all* the time!

"Anyone can do something by accident," said Dan. "If you wet when you're sleeping sometimes, it will be just a silly old accident.

"You won't feel bad, because you'll know that fewer and fewer accidents are going to happen, until they won't happen at all, ever."

"Oh, I want to be dry all night so much!" said Christopher. "I hate wetting when I'm sleeping. I want to be the boss over my bladder muscle!"

"Of course you do," said Dan. "*Clouds* are supposed to have water come out of them at night — not *you*.

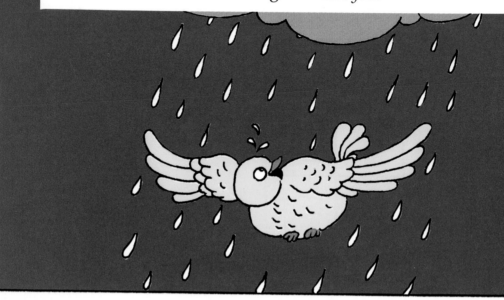

"You don't want to wet when you're asleep. It makes your bed *cold*.

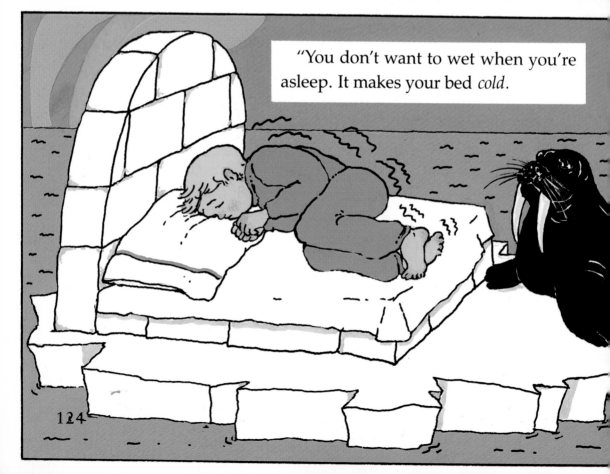

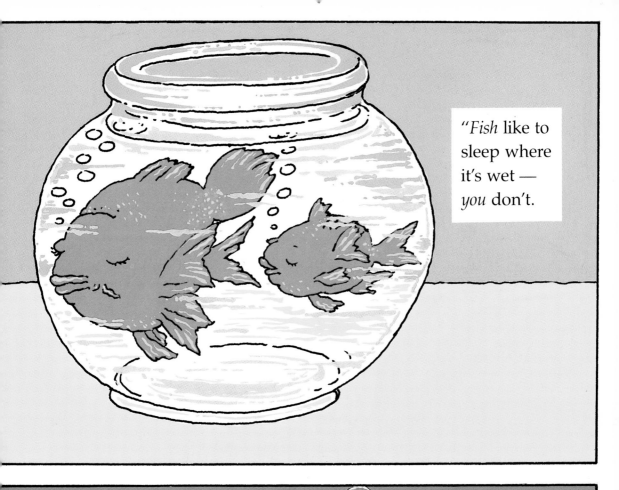

"*Fish* like to sleep where it's wet — *you* don't.

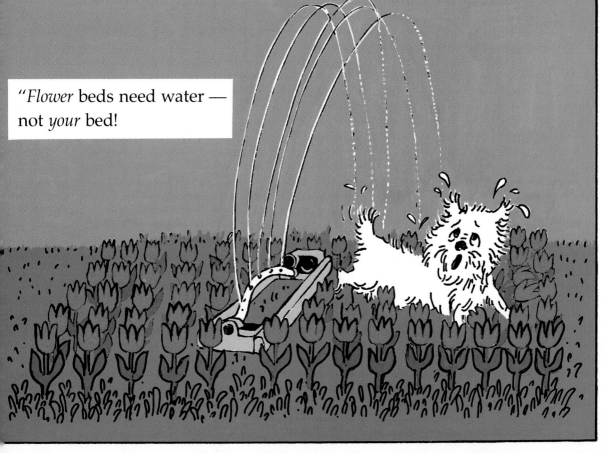

"*Flower* beds need water — not *your* bed!

"You're going to be dry all night very soon," said Dan.

"Really?" said Christopher.

"Of course," said Dan. "You don't think ALIENS wet when they're sleeping, do you?"

Christopher laughed. "I guess not."

"And ROBOTS are dry all night, aren't they?" said Dan.

"They've got to be," laughed Christopher. "Otherwise they'd rust!"

"And all the MONSTERS I know are dry all night," said Dan. "It would be *horrible* for a monster to wet when it was sleeping."

Christopher smiled. "I guess if aliens and robots and monsters can be dry all night, *kids* can be dry all night, too!"

"Of course they can," said Dan.

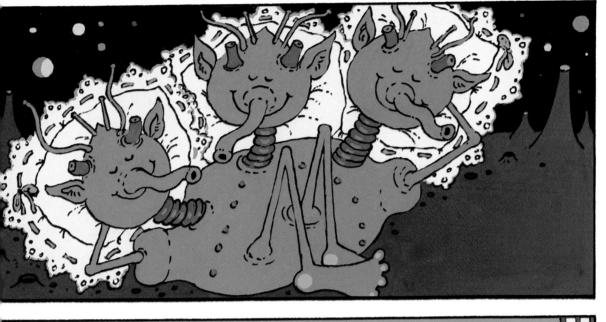

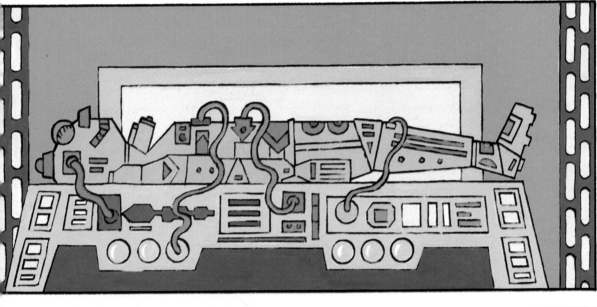

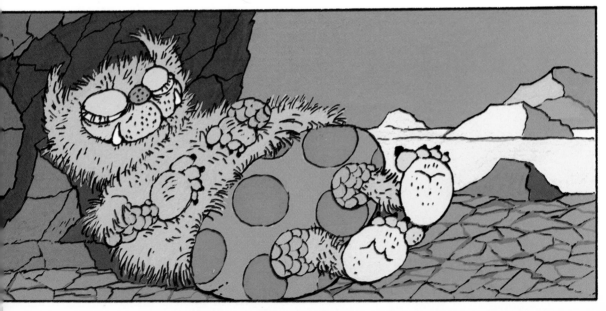

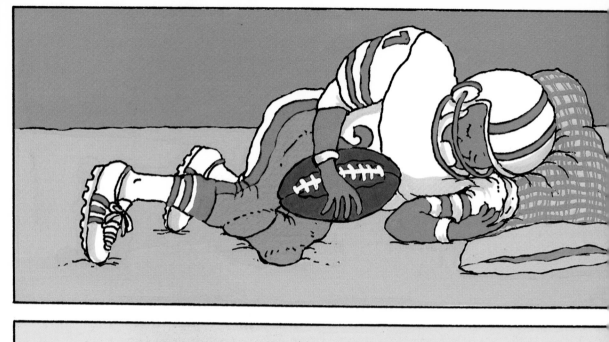

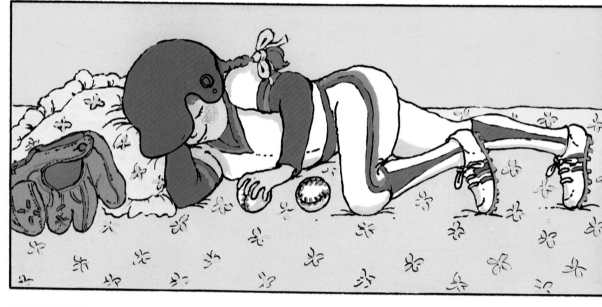

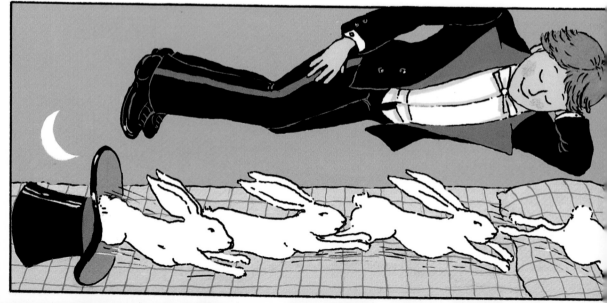

"KIDS WHO PLAY FOOTBALL used to wet when they were sleeping — but now they're dry all night.

"KIDS WHO PLAY BASEBALL used to wet when they were sleeping — but now they're dry all night.

"KIDS WHO PUT ON MAGIC SHOWS used to wet when they were sleeping — but now they're dry all night.

"Soon you're going to be dry all night, just like them," said Dan.

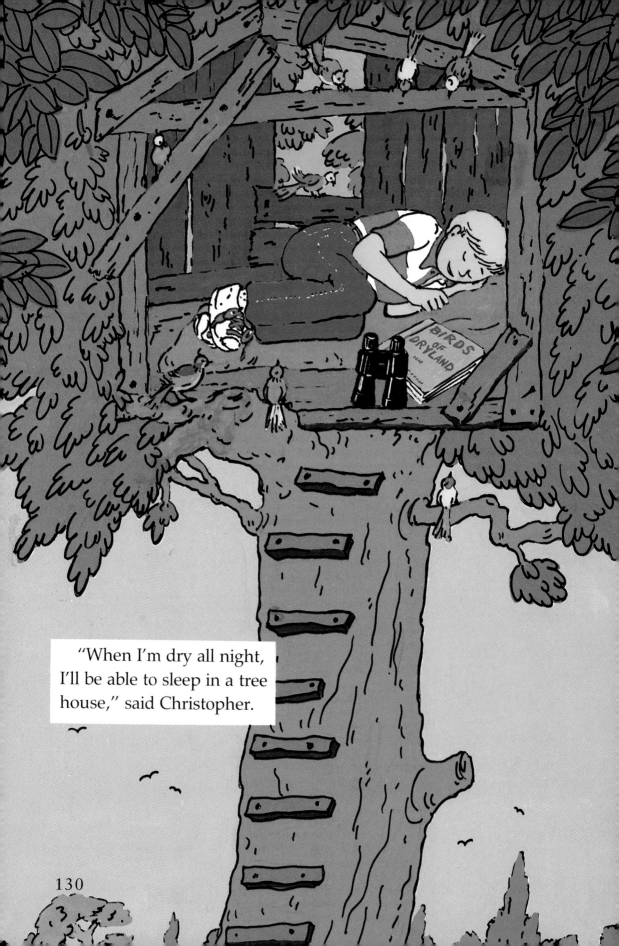

"When I'm dry all night, I'll be able to sleep in a tree house," said Christopher.

130

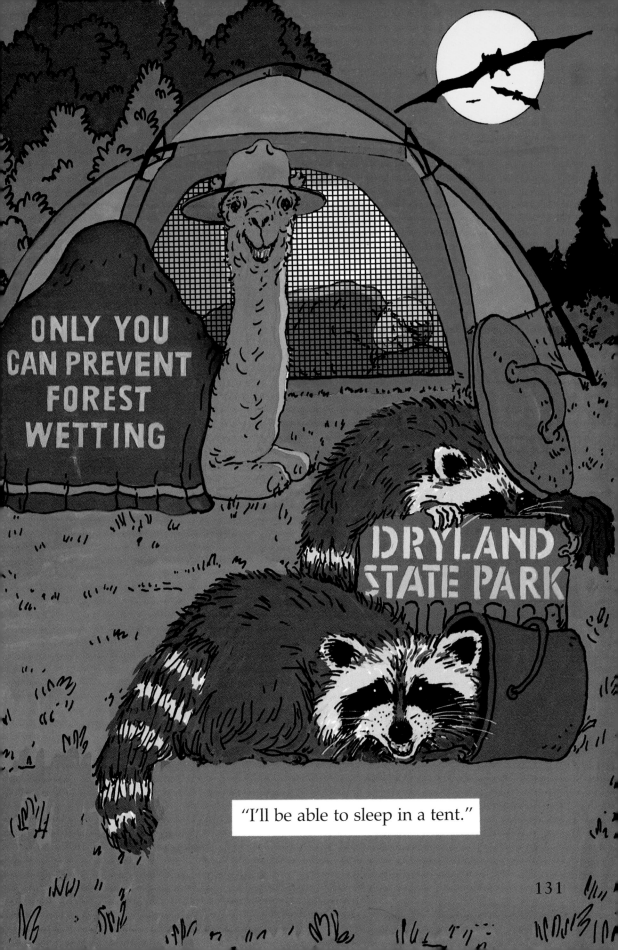

"I'll be able to sleep in a tent."

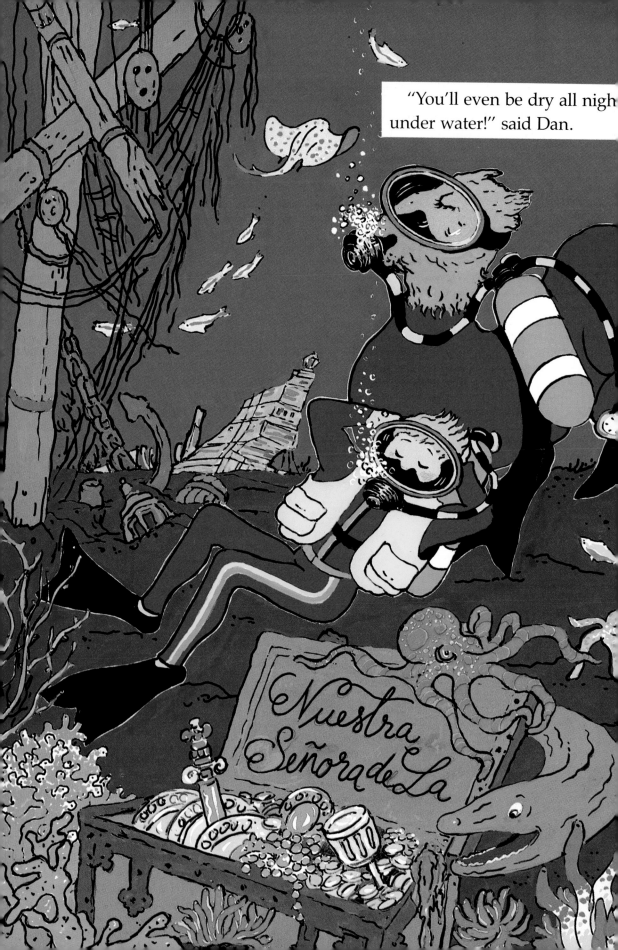

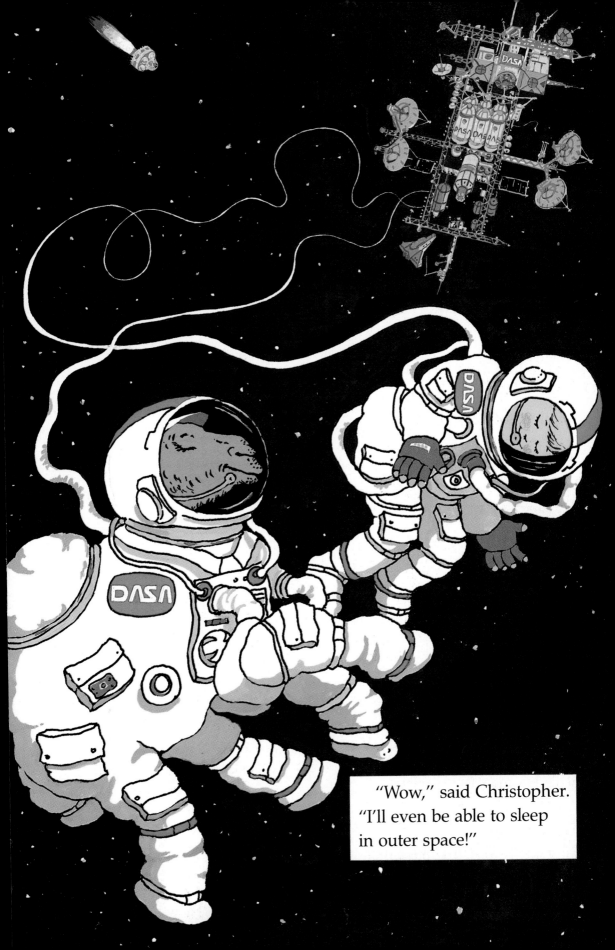

"Wow," said Christopher. "I'll even be able to sleep in outer space!"

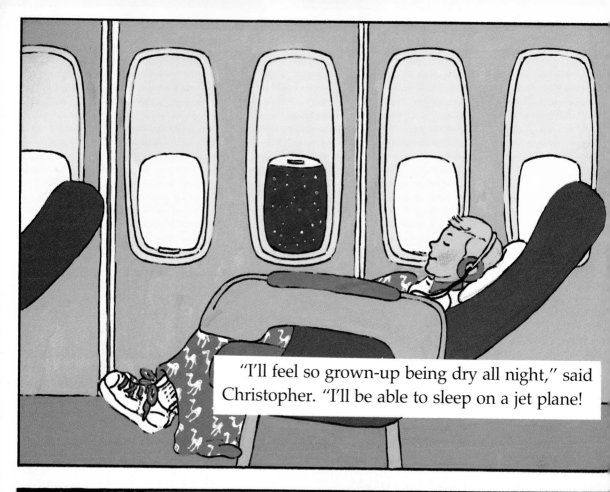

"I'll feel so grown-up being dry all night," said Christopher. "I'll be able to sleep on a jet plane!

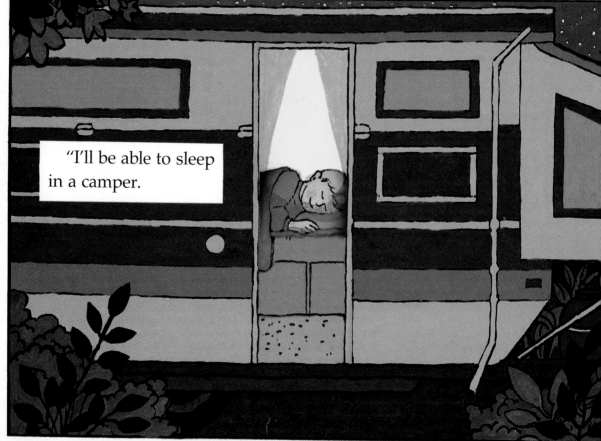

"I'll be able to sleep in a camper.

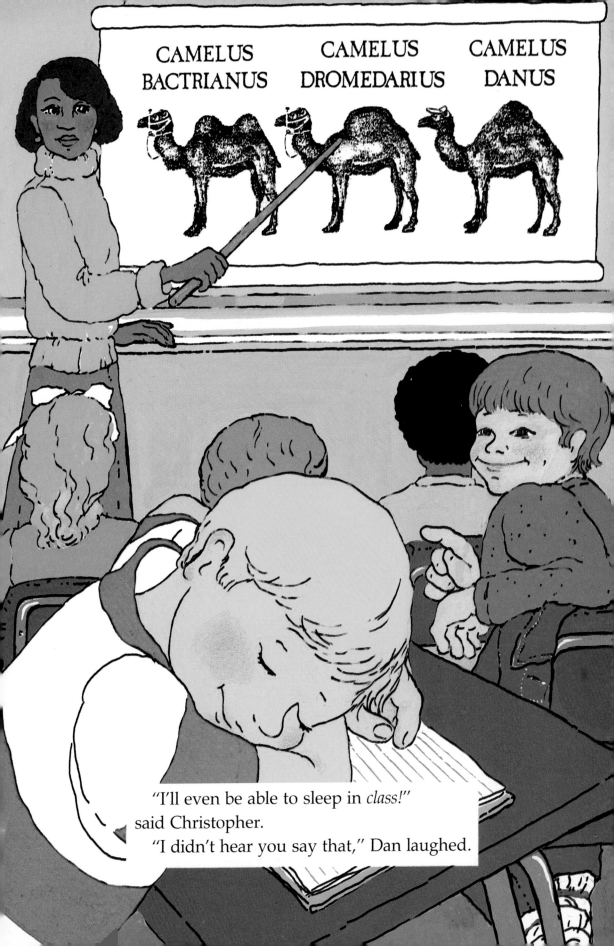

"I'll even be able to sleep in *class!*"
said Christopher.
"I didn't hear you say that," Dan laughed.

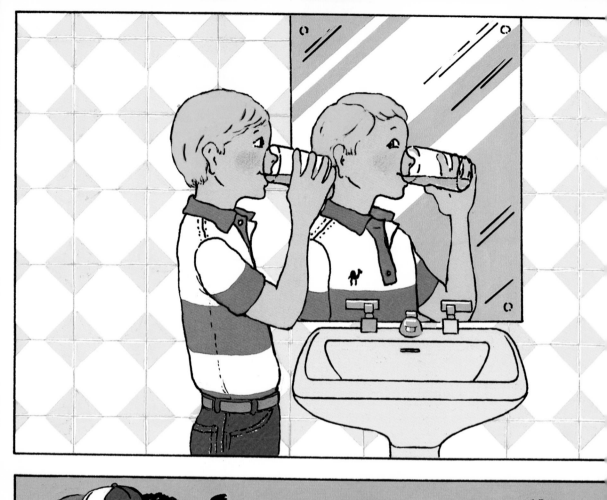

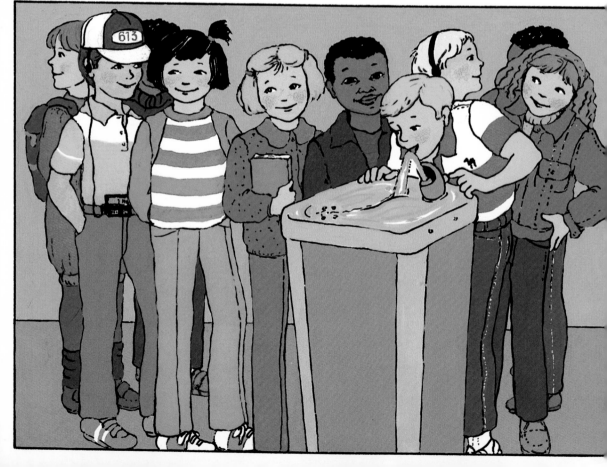

Nobody had to remind Christopher to drink plenty of powerful H_2O all day to help him be dry all night. He hated wetting when he was sleeping, and he really wanted to stop. He knew it was his job to do the things he needed to do to be dry all night.

Christopher drank H_2O at school. He drank H_2O at his friends' houses. He drank H_2O at home. He drank H_2O everywhere.

After Christopher ate supper, he didn't drink anything unless he felt pretty thirsty.

All day long, Christopher listened to what his bladder muscle was telling him. When his bladder muscle felt like it was all filled up with urine, he stopped whatever he was doing and went into the bathroom and put the urine in the toilet, where he wanted it to go.

Every afternoon, Christopher drank a great big glass of H_2O. Then he went into his bedroom and closed the door. He turned off all the lights except for one light near his bed. Then he read his *Dry All Night* book and saw the pictures inside his head.

First Christopher saw a picture inside his head of himself on the Fire Chief Ride.

When Christopher was seeing the picture inside his head, he told himself, "If my bladder muscle gets all filled up with urine when I'm sleeping, it can just stay full, all night long, without any urine going out.

"Or, the full feeling will wake me up right away, just like a fire bell ringing really, really loud.

"As soon as I wake up, I'll walk into the bathroom and put the urine in the toilet, where I want it to go."

Christopher felt really good, because he was going to be the boss over his bladder muscle all day long and all night long, just the way a fire chief is the boss over his fire truck all day long and all night long.

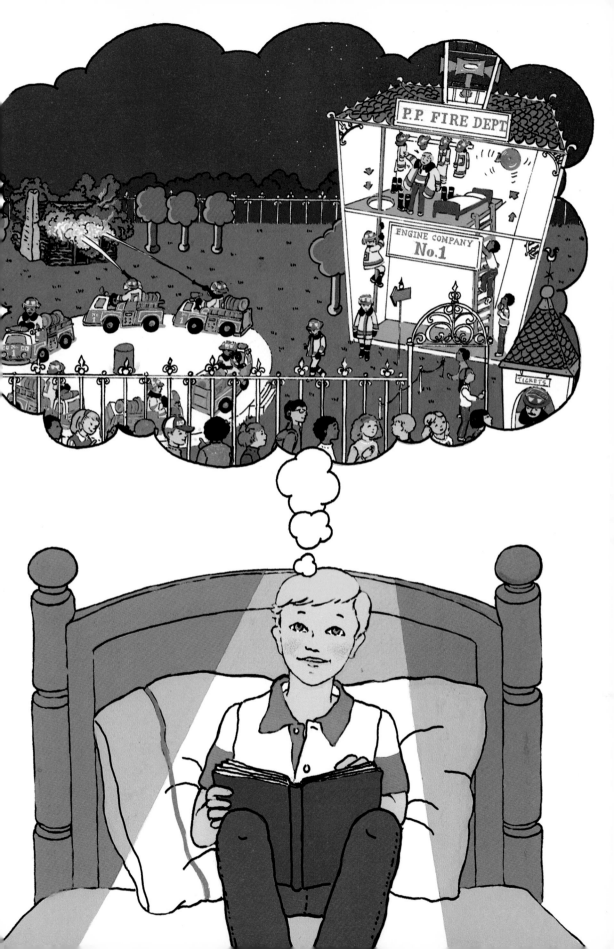

Then, Christopher saw another picture inside his head. He saw a picture of himself getting out of bed because the feeling of his bladder muscle being all filled up was like a fire bell ringing really, really loud, waking him right up so that he could walk to the bathroom.

Christopher made believe that he was waking up because his bladder muscle was all filled up with urine.

When Christopher was seeing the picture inside his head, he told himself, "Urine will only go out of my bladder muscle when I'm wide awake. If my bladder muscle gets all filled up with urine when I'm sleeping, it can just stay full, all night long, without any urine going out.

"Or, the full feeling will be like a fire bell ringing really, really loud, waking me right up."

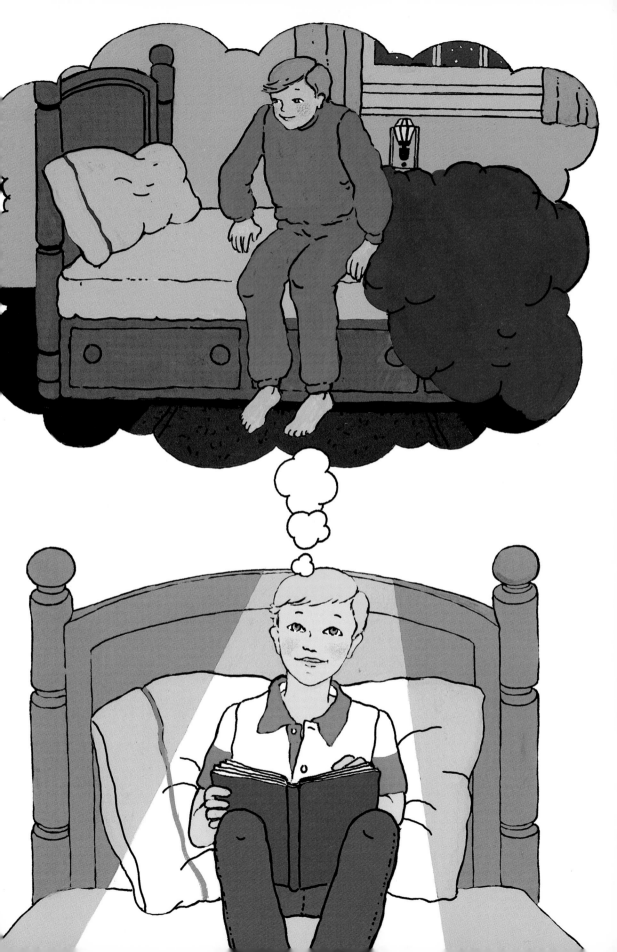

Then, Christopher saw a picture inside his head of himself in the bathroom, urinating into the toilet.

Christopher made believe that he woke right up when his bladder muscle felt like it was all filled up with urine. He made believe that he walked into the bathroom. He made believe that he was putting the urine in the toilet, where he wanted it to go.

Christopher felt really good about putting the urine in the toilet, because he was the boss over his bladder muscle, just like the fire chief is the boss over his fire truck.

When Christopher was seeing the picture inside his head, just like it was a TV picture, he told himself, "As soon as I get back in my bed, I'll fall asleep right away."

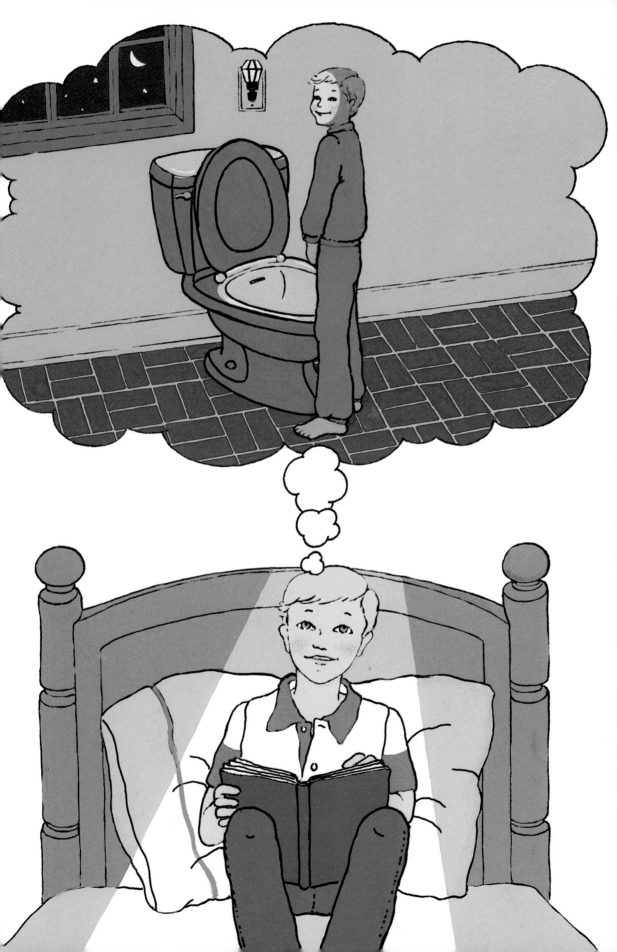

Then, Christopher saw a picture inside his head of himself sleeping in his dry bed.

When Christopher was seeing the picture inside his head, he told his bladder muscle that if it gets filled up with urine, it can just stay full, without any urine going out.

He told himself, "Soon I'm going to be able to sleep all night long, every night, without any urine going out of my bladder muscle."

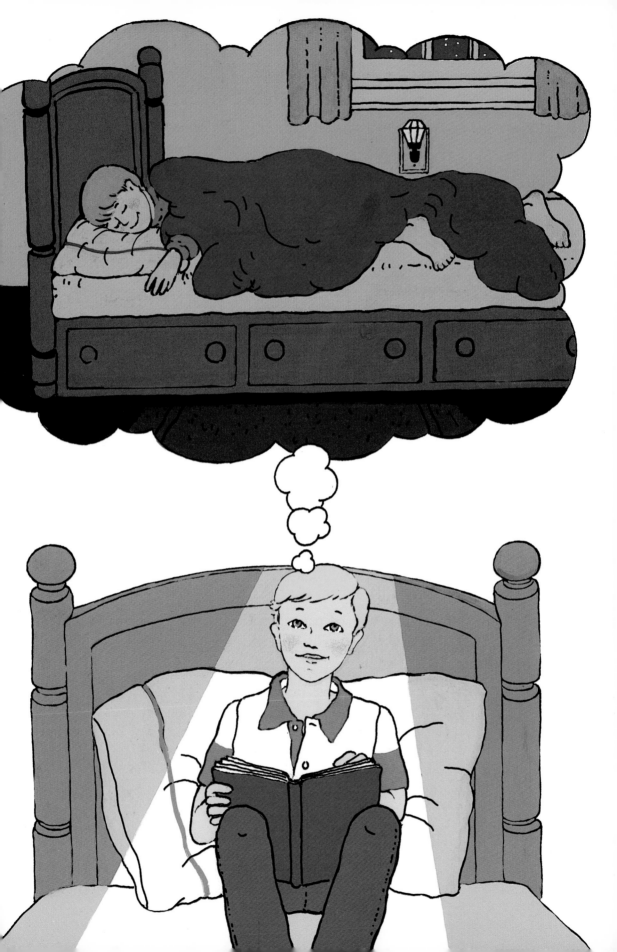

Then, Christopher saw a picture inside his head of himself waking up in the morning after he was dry all night. He felt so nice and dry, it was as if he'd been sleeping in a desert, where it's dry all the time.

Christopher made believe that he didn't wet when he was sleeping.

He made believe that he felt really, really good because he was the boss over his bladder muscle when he was sleeping.

Every afternoon, Christopher sat on his bed and read his *Dry All Night* book and saw the pictures inside his head, one after another.

He had fun reading his book and seeing the pictures inside his head, because he knew he was doing the things he needed to do to be the boss over his bladder muscle, all by himself.

After he saw the pictures inside his head and finished reading his book, he went into the bathroom and urinated into the toilet.

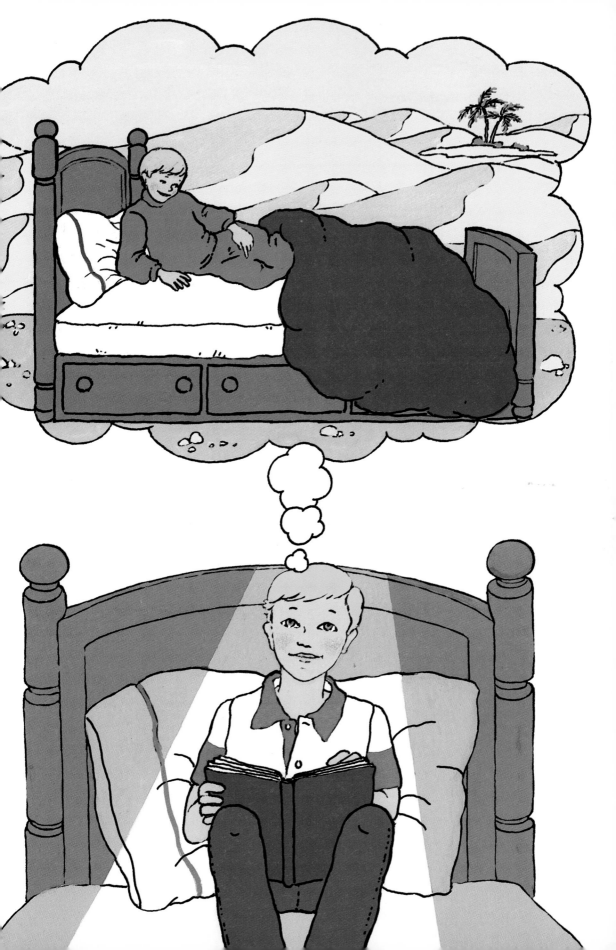

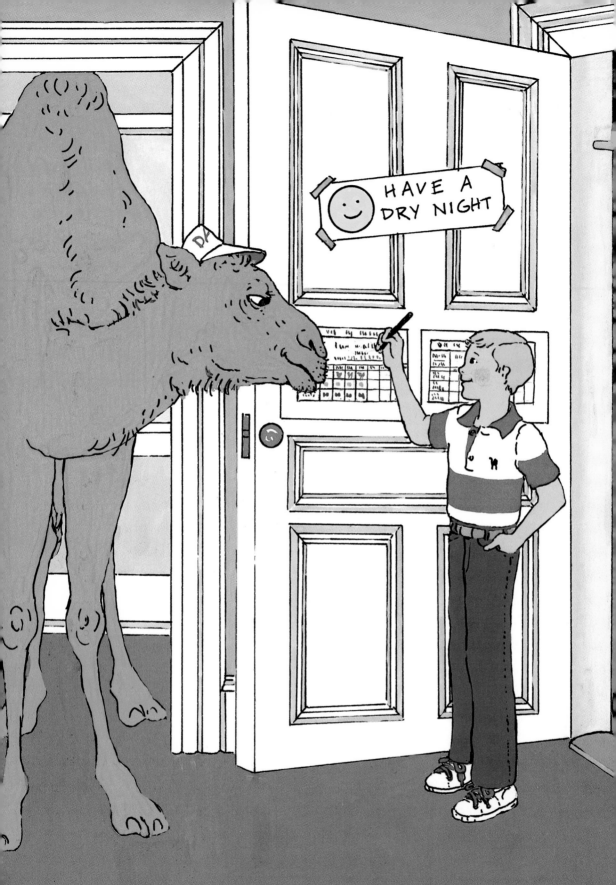

"I want you to hang up your Dry All Night scoreboard where nobody can see it but you," said Dan. "Then you'll fill it in."

Every day, Christopher drew a glass on his scoreboard to show that he drank a great big glass of H_2O.

Every day, he drew a book on his scoreboard to show that he read his book and saw the pictures inside his head of himself being the boss over his bladder muscle.

And whenever he woke up and found out that he didn't wet when he was sleeping, he drew a picture of Dan the Magic Camel to show that he was dry all night.

After he ate supper, Christopher didn't drink too much. After supper he didn't drink any H_2O, or milk, or juice, or soda, unless he was pretty thirsty. He knew that not drinking too much after supper would help him to be dry all night.

Christopher never drank anything at all right before he went to sleep. Every night, just before he got into bed, he went into the bathroom and urinated. He turned on his little light in the bathroom so it would stay on all night long.

Then he turned off all the lights in his bedroom except for one little light. Then he sat down on his bed and saw the pictures inside his head.

Every night, right before Christopher went to sleep, he put his *Dry All Night* book under his pillow, so that he would remember to be dry all night.

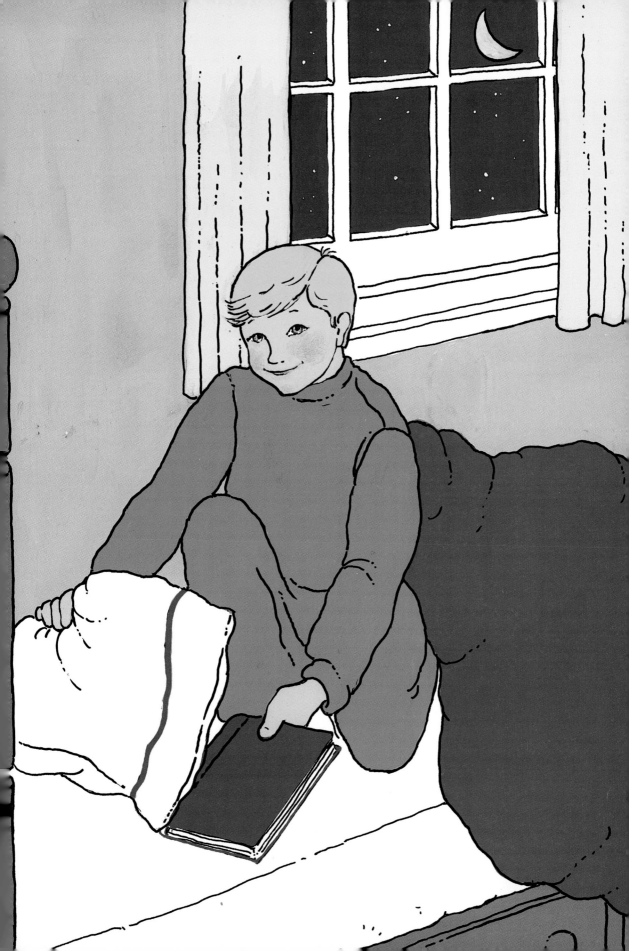

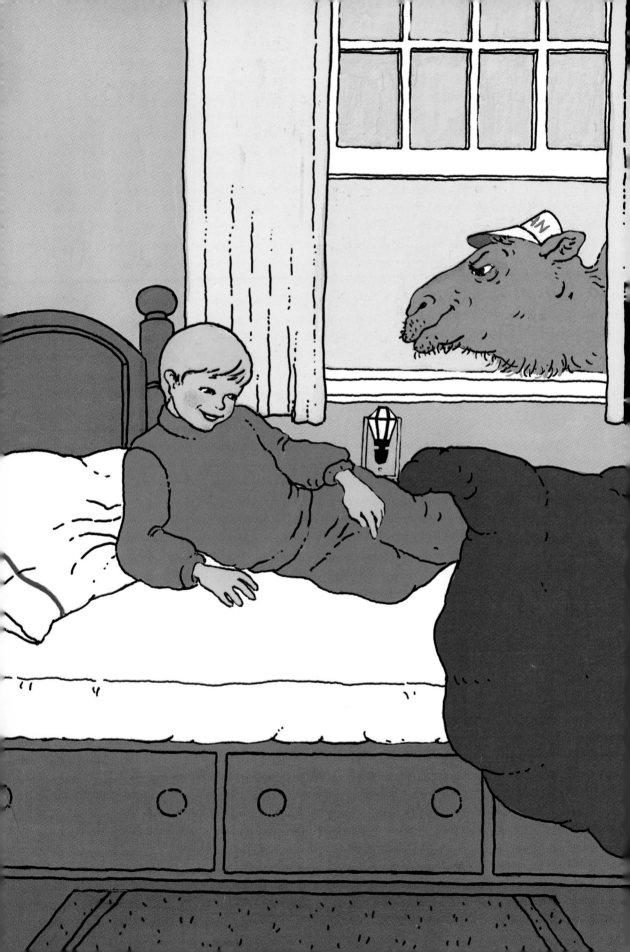

Christopher liked the feeling of waking up in the morning in a nice dry bed. He liked the feeling of doing special things all by himself to become dry all night. He liked the feeling of being the boss over his bladder muscle.

Soon Christopher was having more and more dry nights. Soon he was drawing more and more pictures of Dan on his Dry All Night scoreboard. Being dry all night made him feel so grown-up!

"Soon I'll be able to sleep all night long without urinating," Christopher told himself.

"I'm really proud of you," said Dan to Christopher. "I'd walk a mile for a kid like you!"

By the time karate camp was about to begin, Christopher was dry all night all the time.

"Thanks for helping me to be dry all night," Christopher said to Dan.

"You don't have to thank me," said Dan. *"You're* the one who did it!"

"Will you come with me to karate camp?" said Christopher. "I'm sure Master Lee wouldn't mind having a magic camel around."

"You've made me very happy," said Dan. "And I'd love to come with you to karate camp. But there are lots of other girls and boys for me to help. I want them to be dry all night too."

"It is good to see you here, Christopher," said Master Lee. "I knew that you would be with us. Come. It is time."

"Goodbye, Dan," said Christopher as he got on the bus. He felt so grown-up going to karate camp. "I'll never forget you."

Christopher had a wonderful summer. He made lots of new friends. He was the junior karate champion of the whole camp.

And best of all, he was dry all night.

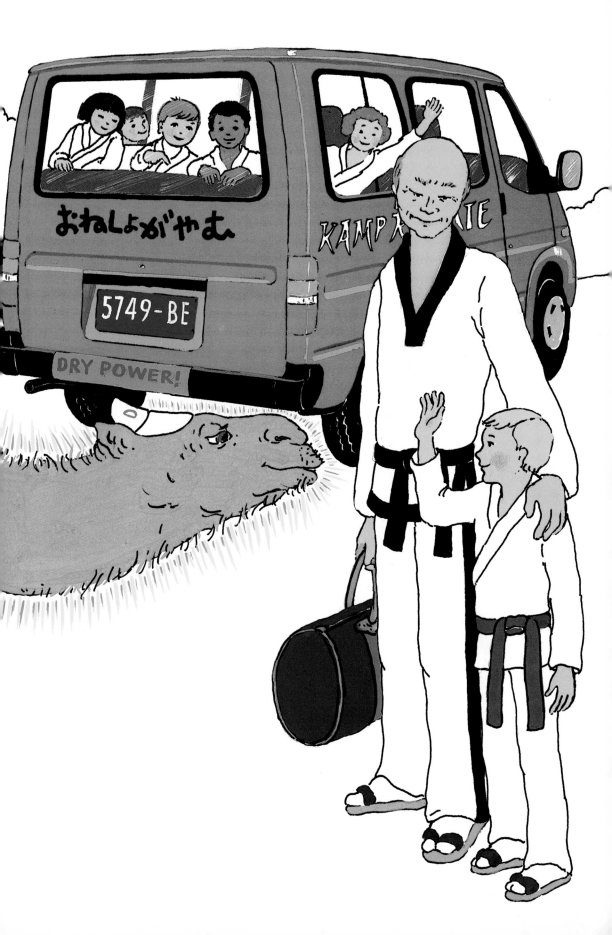

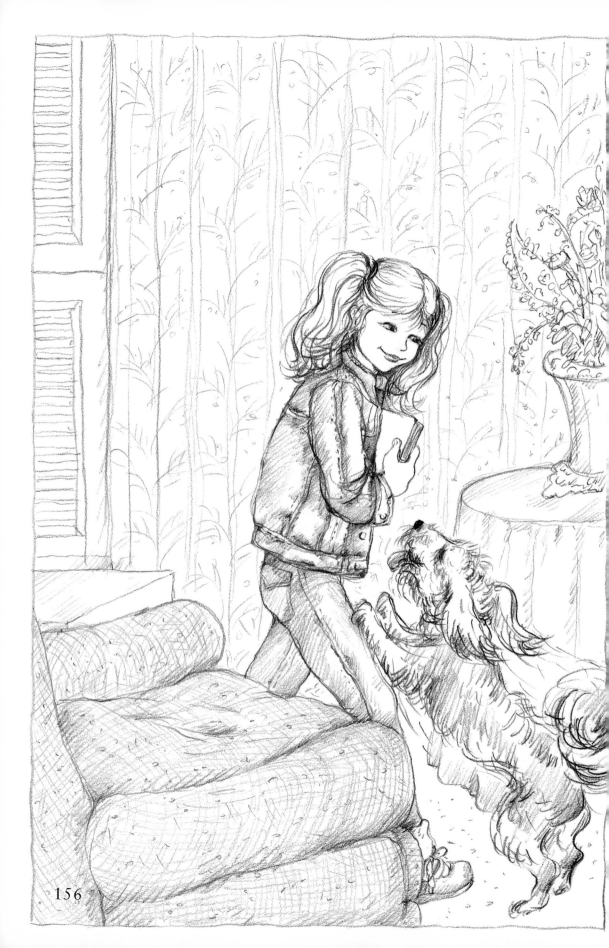

Erin had fun reading her book. She enjoyed seeing Christopher do easy things all by himself to become dry all night.

She decided to read her book every day, and to do everything Christopher did.

Nobody had to remind Erin to do the things she wanted to do to be dry all night.

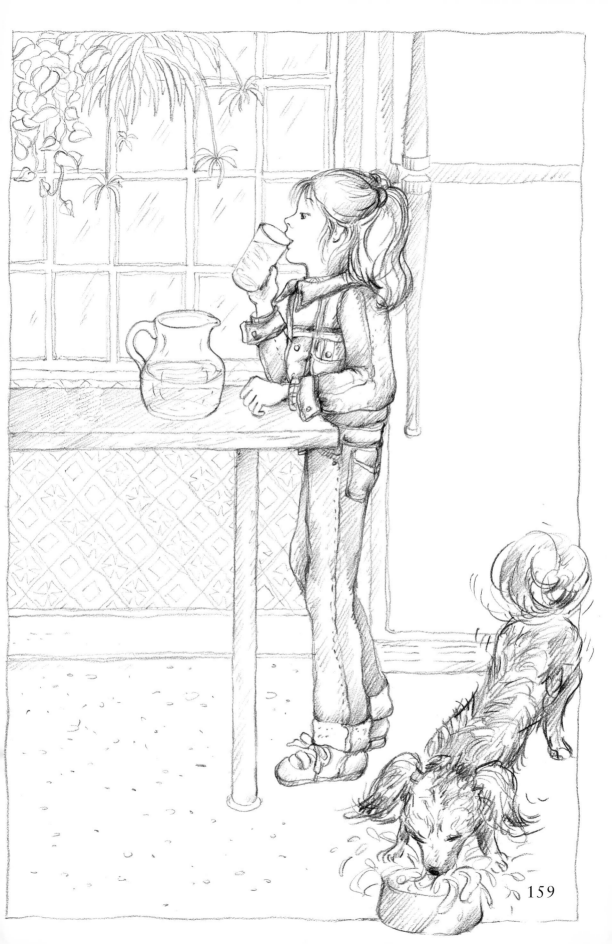

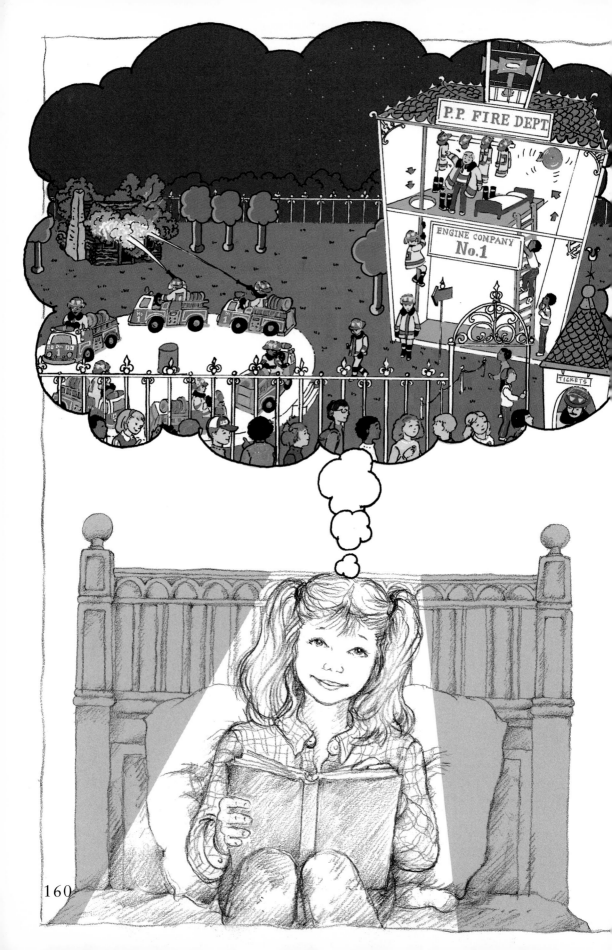

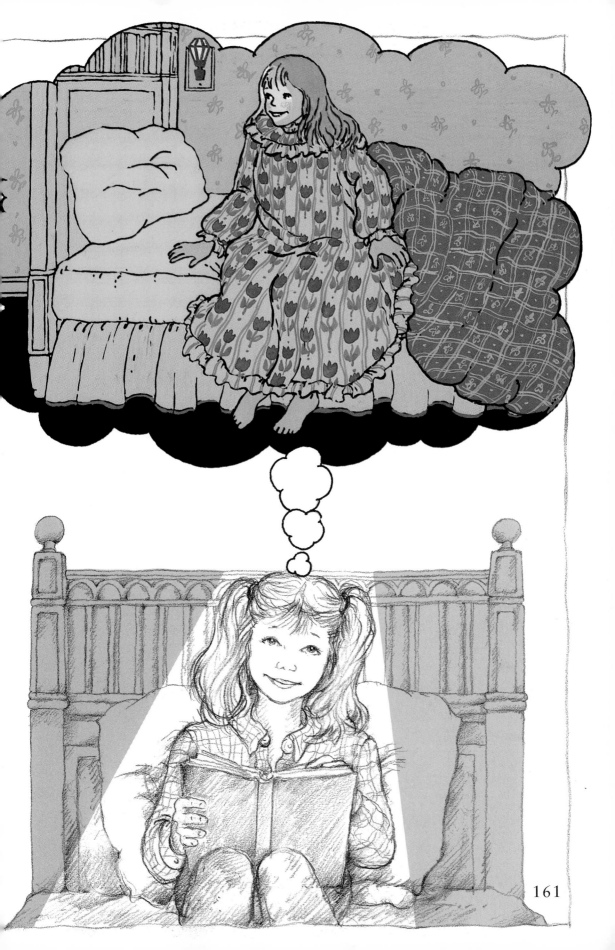

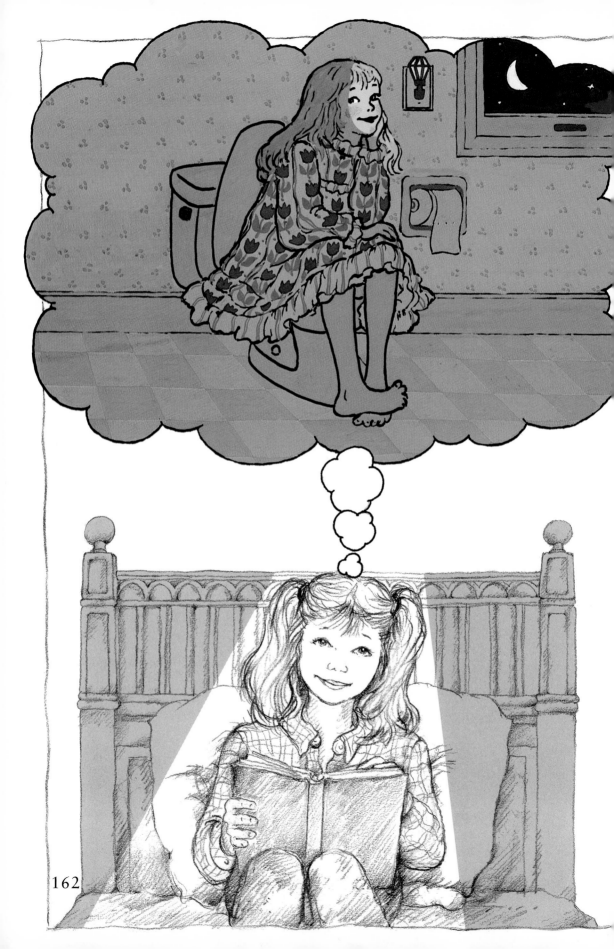

162

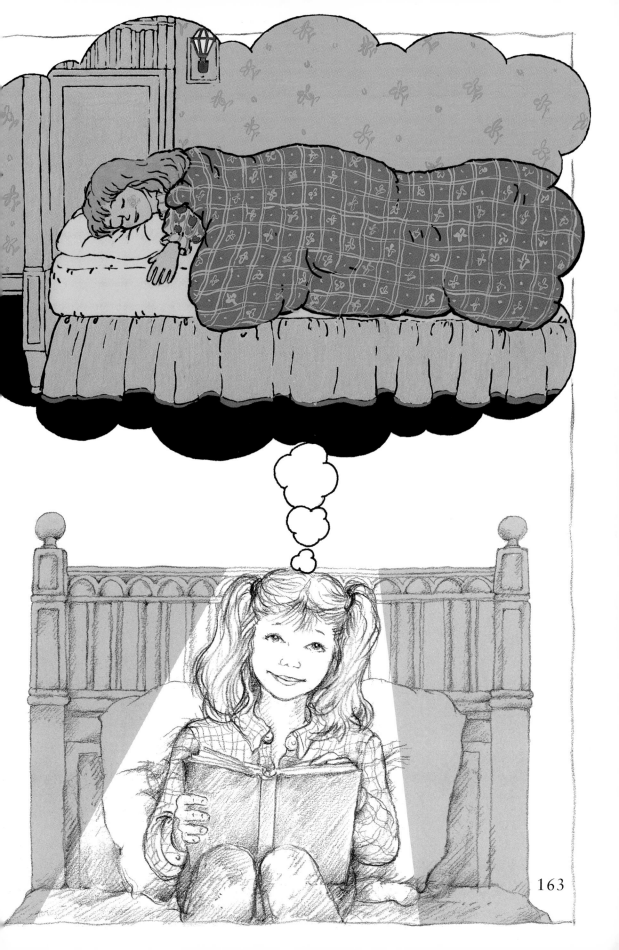

163

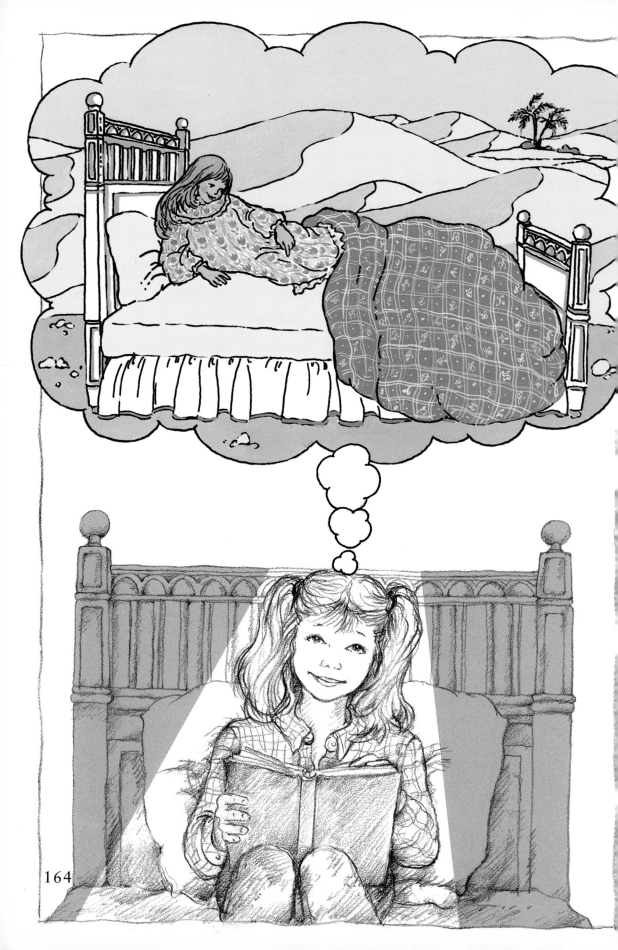

Erin had fun seeing the pictures inside her head. After she saw the pictures she went into the bathroom and urinated into the toilet.

When Erin went to sleep with her book under her pillow, she felt that she was going to be dry all night.

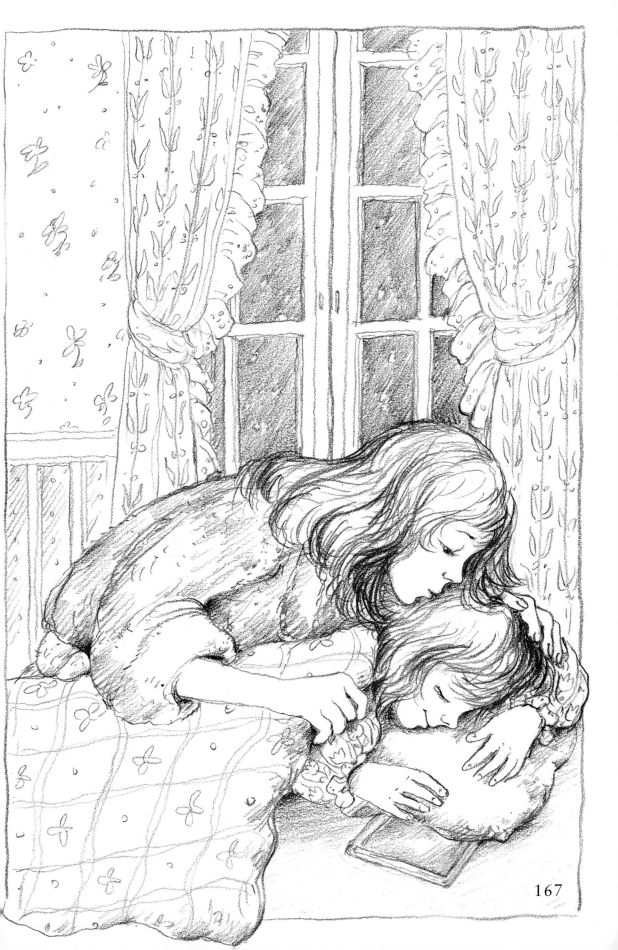

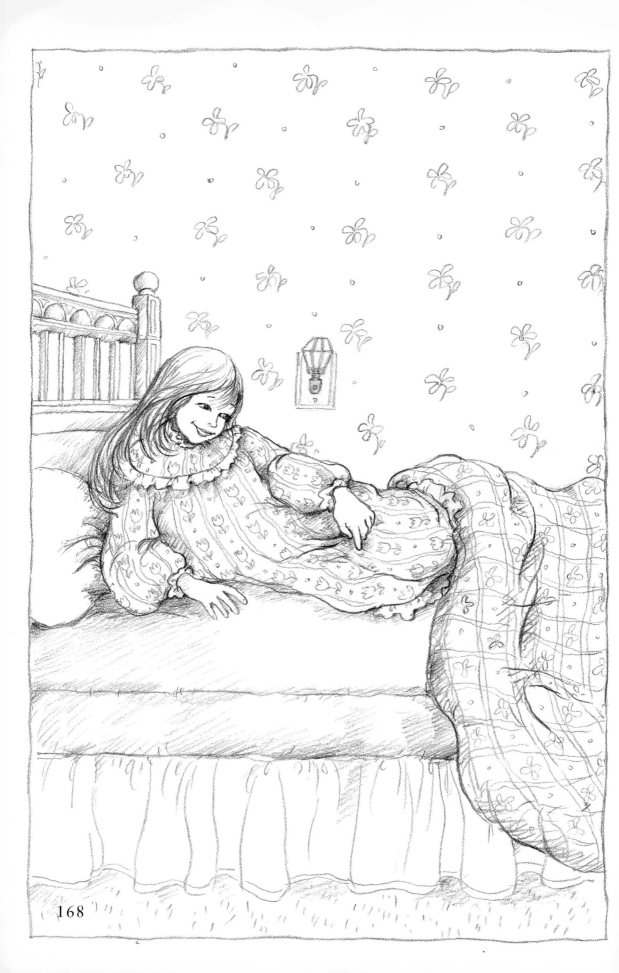

Erin felt really grown-up doing the things she needed to do to be dry all night, all by herself.

• She drank plenty of powerful H_2O all day.
• Every afternoon, she drank a great big glass of H_2O. Then she sat on her bed and read her book and saw the pictures inside her head of herself being the boss over her bladder muscle. When she was seeing the pictures, she told herself, "When my bladder muscle gets all filled up with urine, it can just stay full, all night long, without any urine going out.

"Or, the full feeling will wake me up right away, just like a fire bell ringing really, really loud. As soon as I wake up, I'll walk to the bathroom and put the urine in the toilet, where I want it to go."
• When she saw the picture inside her head of herself waking up after she was dry all night, she told herself, "Soon I'll be able to sleep all night long, every night, without any urine going out of my bladder muscle."
• After she saw the pictures, she felt good, and she went into her bathroom and urinated into the toilet.
• After she ate supper she didn't drink anything unless she felt pretty thirsty. She didn't drink anything at all right before she went to sleep.
• Right before she went to sleep, she went into the bathroom and urinated into the toilet. Then she sat on her bed and saw the pictures inside her head again.
• She kept her book under her pillow when she was sleeping, so she'd remember to be dry all night.

Soon Erin didn't wet when she was sleeping. She was dry all night.

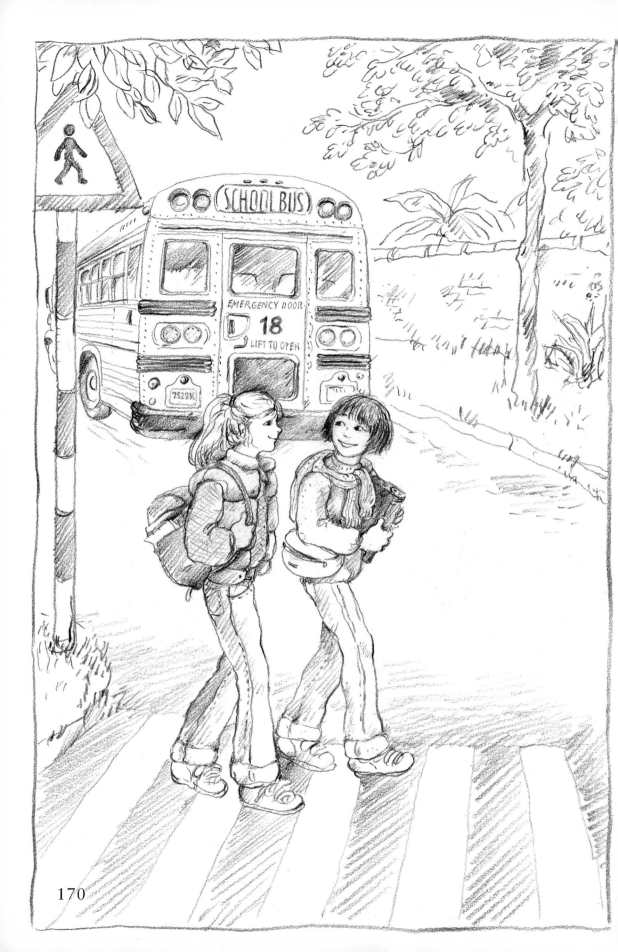

One day, Brandi said to Erin, "I sure do wish you'd sleep over at my house some time."

"Okay," said Erin. "How about tonight?"

"Can you really?" said Brandi. Brandi was so happy. She liked Erin so much. She thought Erin was so smart and so pretty. "Will your mom let you?"

"Of course she will," said Erin. Erin felt so good knowing she wouldn't wet when she was sleeping at Brandi's house.

Erin went to Brandi's house to sleep over. Erin and Brandi ate together. They made a get-well card together for a friend who was sick. They watched TV together. They even played together after they were supposed to be in bed.

"I've wanted you to sleep over for such a long time," whispered Brandi. "Whenever I asked you and you said no, I was so unhappy."

"My mom wouldn't let me until tonight," whispered Erin. "But from now on, she's going to let me sleep over whenever I want."

"That's great," said Brandi. "Because I'd like to have you sleep over all the time. Like maybe once every month."

"I've got an idea," said Erin. "Why don't *you* come and sleep over at *my* house next month?!"

"Well, gee . . ." said Brandi.

"And the month after that, I'll come here," Erin said. "And the next month, you'll sleep over at my house."

"I don't know," said Brandi.

"What do you mean, 'you don't know'?" said Erin.

"Maybe I won't be able to," said Brandi.

"Why not?" asked Erin.

"I don't think my mom will let me," said Brandi.

"Why won't she?" said Erin.

And then Erin had an idea . . .

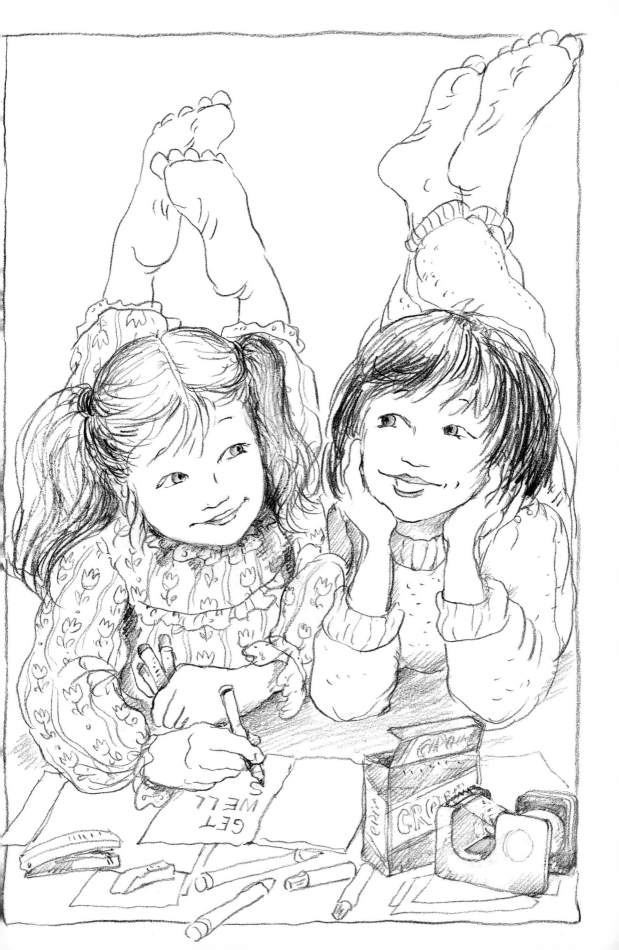

"Hey," said Erin. "Don't tell me *you* wet when you're sleeping!"

"What makes you think I do?" said Brandi.

"Because that's why *I* couldn't sleep over before," said Erin. "Because I used to wet when I was asleep!"

"You're kidding," said Brandi.

"Would I kid about something like *that*?" said Erin.

"But you said —"

"I know," said Erin. "I said it was my mom. But it was true. How could I ask her, if I knew I was going to wet when I was asleep? Is that why *your* mom won't let you sleep at *my* house?"

"Oh!" said Brandi. "You guessed my secret. I *do* wet when I'm sleeping! I do!" And Brandi started to cry.

"Come on," said Erin. "Don't cry."

"Why not?" Brandi sobbed. "It's *terrible!*"

"No, it isn't," said Erin. "Lots of kids wet when they're sleeping. It's nothing to be ashamed of. Look — we didn't want to tell each other. So each of us thought we were the only one who wet in the whole world! Wasn't that silly?"

Brandi stopped crying. She felt a lot better.

"I've got an idea," said Erin. "I'll tell my mom that you wet when you're sleeping. She'll talk to your mom, and your mom will get you the book that helped me. Your mom will give the book to you as a present.

"You'll have fun reading it. It'll tell you what you need to do to stop wetting when you're asleep. You'll be able to do the things it tells you to do all by yourself. You'll do everything the book says. And soon you'll be —

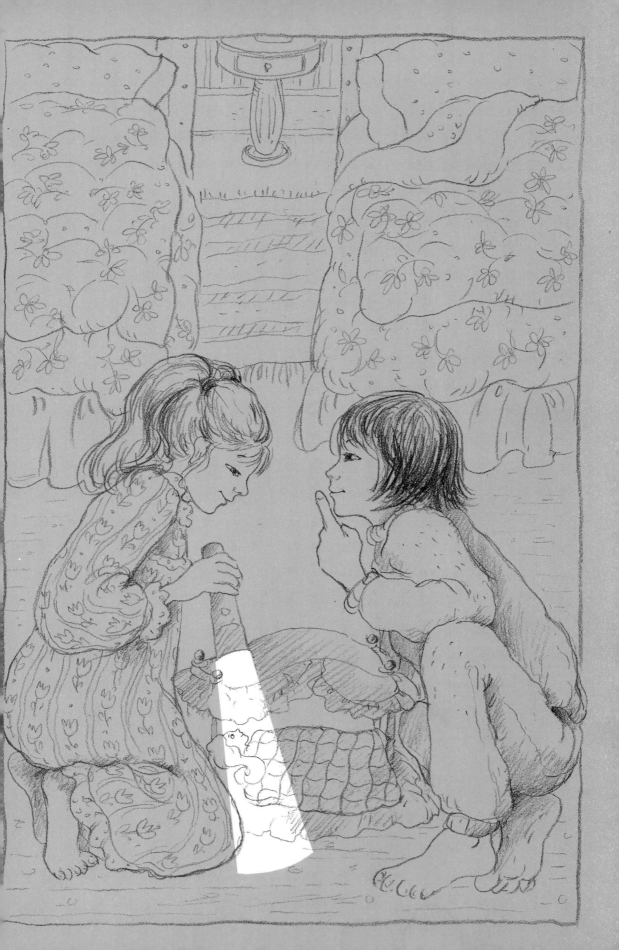

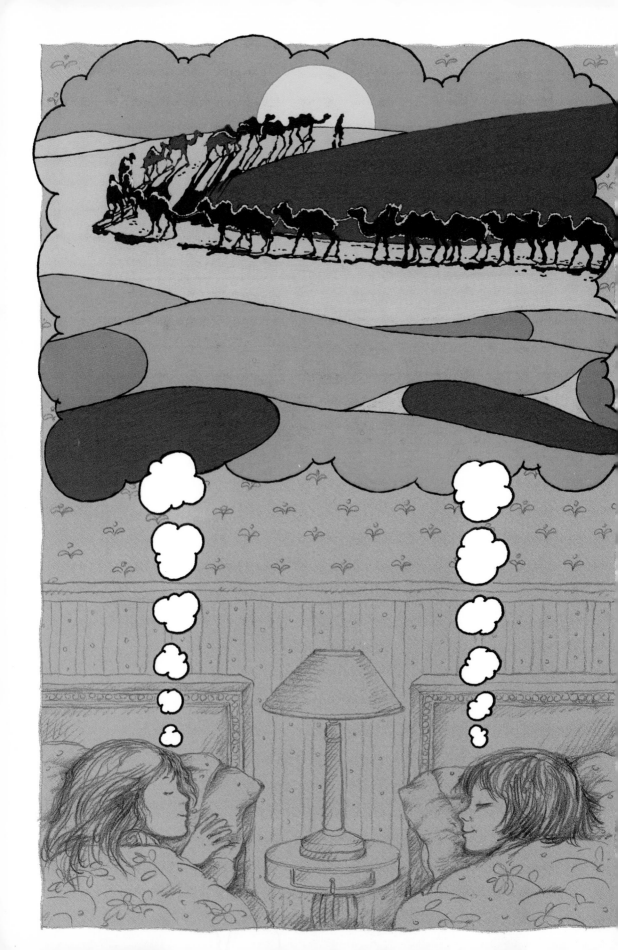

Dry All Night.